Rejuvenat

By Dr. Ya

Eight Steps to Perfect Health

Information
and
Instructions

Koyfman Center for Health and Rejuvenation

The Great War Inside You

When toxins come to a body,
the immune system begins
to fight them.
In counterattack, the toxins
link up with their best friends,
the parasites,
and use their most dangerous weapon,
poison.
This constant war leaves
the immune system tired and weak
and opens the door to diseases.
Killing the parasites and
cleansing the body from toxins
releases the immune system from its
major enemies.
The immune system becomes stronger
and health returns.

Preface

This book is published, not as a substitute for, but as a supplement to the supervision of a professional healthcare practitioner. The procedures described in this book are designed to support the body's immune system through internal cleansing so the body can heal itself and experience maximum vitality. They are preventative in nature for the improvement of human health. They are also designed to provide a greater self-awareness of personal health.

This book is not intended to provide medical consultation, diagnostic services, prognostication, health-related suggestions or recommendations, treatment procedures, or prescription of remedies for any ailment or condition. The author of this book does not treat any disease or provide any cure.

Because each person is unique, the author encourages each reader to pursue a daily self-care program tailored to his or her particular situation, based on that person's own best evaluation of the circumstances.

Koyfman's Center for Health and Rejuvenation, Inc.
300 Merchant Drive, Suite 304
Norcross, GA 30093
(770) 908-2305
www.koyfmancenter.com

Contents

Prologue:

How to Use This Book

This book describes the techniques and philosophy that make up "Deep Internal Body Cleansing." This powerful suite of procedures is designed to help remove harmful toxins (chemical, biological, and mental) from specific organs and systems in your body. Once these disease-causing toxins are fully purged from the body, **maximum health is an attainable goal and a sustainable lifestyle.**

How to Use the Information

As you delve into each of the cleansing techniques recorded here you will find instructions on how to prepare and what to expect, what your part is and what the Center does. For example, as toxins are gently flushed from the body, some people sometimes experience minor discomfort as these toxins pass through the body on the way out. This discomfort is very temporary, but its possibility is important to know in order to understand "what's happening."

This book also provides information on what to eat to support your newly increased health.

Please read the instructions carefully, as they are vital to the success of these procedures. Do not skip any part of the instructions, and certainly do not neglect the whole of any one of them. It is recommended that you read each set of instructions several times to be sure you understand it correctly. Then either highlight or make notes of the basics of each step so you can remember what you have learned.

Please remember that the **"Trinity of Good Health"** is more than (1) eating correctly, (2) exercising properly, and (3) flushing toxins from the body. The Trinity of Good Health includes that most powerful of alliances: (1) correct knowledge, (2) a trained and experienced health care provider to guide you in the techniques, and (3) YOU.

Never underestimate the importance *you* play in all of this. It is not enough to merely "show up" for the procedures. You want to engage the knowledge you have and marry it to a focused commitment. When the power of the mind and the commitment of the heart are brought into play, all of the other elements of good health are given their greatest strength.

If you ignore the part you have to play (especially following the instructions) then results can be greatly diminished.

How to Use the Herbs, Beverages, and Solutions

All solutions which we use at the Center are completely organic, and made by hand by professionals for each individual. These solutions are made from fresh juices, herbs, minerals, and purified water.

All cleansings performed with these solutions require special preparation, and are based on knowledge acquired from centuries of practice. Professional experience and training are critical to the correct administration of these solutions to yield the maximum healing effect.

The contents of each of these solutions used at the Center, plus the techniques for properly blending the solutions, are proprietary information and are the intellectual property of the Center. Trying to duplicate these solutions at home can yield results that either interfere with or prove counterproductive to the cleansing procedures. Trying to fake these solutions can even be harmful since there are critical synergies involved with the components of the solutions.

Introduction:

Health and Cleansing

Healing through cleansing procedures is the easiest, quickest, and most natural way to get your health back. Cleansing is the best way, not only to heal problems, but also to prevent illness and maintain good health.

Cleansing

The most basic and undeniable concept in the health of the human organism is that "foreign" materials (things that were never meant to be part of the body) do **not** increase health. In fact, foreign objects *in any working system* (including mechanical) interfere with its proper functioning. (Scatter a handful of nuts, bolts and washers in the crankcase of an automobile and see what you get.)

The equivalent is true of our bodies. Unnatural chemicals and unwelcome biological agents (colds and flu, for example) interfere with the proper functioning of organs and systems, and use up the valuable resources of the immune system. Getting rid of these toxins paves the way for healing and prevention of illnesses.

Recently, many people have begun to understand this idea, and to popularize words like "cleansing," "detox," "detoxification," and other similar words and phrases. Each of these descriptions is partially true, but the real cleansing of the organism is something very different and a lot more effective.

The real internal cleansing uses the same concept that works for external cleansing. Think about it. To wash away dirt from the outside of your body, you use a lot of running water with solvents. The water carries the solvents to the area needing cleaning, and then carries the dirt away. The solvents dissolve the dirt or make it easier to remove.

For internal cleansing, you still need a lot of clean, purified water in combination with solvents. Solvents for internal cleansing are specific minerals, herbs, fresh juices, chlorophyl, sea salt, natural oils, etc. In some cases, we use solutions that have carefully chosen magnetic characteristics.

As these solutions travel through the digestive tract, they draw toxins out of the tissues. They also dissolve toxins. They act first on the digestive tract and then on other organs like the liver, gall bladder, pancreas, lungs, branchiae, lymph system, etc. For the most successful results, before each cleansing procedure, we recommend a specific preparation which includes gently heating the body and drinking juices, water, herbs, etc.

Because the digestive tract is the major eliminating channel through which we can cleanse almost all the internal organs, all our cleansing procedures finish with either a Colon Cleansing or, better yet, a Whole Digestive System Cleansing [©].

Why Is It Important to Keep the Digestive Tract Clean?

The digestive system is the "kitchen" of the human body in that it provides the food or nutrients our bodies need to live. How we keep that kitchen determines whether we will be feeding ourselves with nutrients or poisoning it with toxins.

Those who are truly interested in maintaining their health know the importance of cleaning the kitchen, as well as the continuing importance of maintaining it by regular cleansings.

No matter how good your diet, in our poisoned world you cannot completely keep toxins out of your body, hence the need for regular cleansings. Toxins not cleansed from the digestive system are absorbed into the blood and lymph systems, spread all over the body, and poison every organ and tissue down to the cellular level.

The immune system, weakened by this toxicity, first grows sluggish and less effective and finally becomes overwhelmed and surrenders. When it collapses, almost every disease can do its worst in your body.

In our Center we utilize a full spectrum of cleansing procedures. One of the simplest and most effective procedures is one I recently created, called "Whole Digestive System Cleansing $^{\circ}$." Our clients like this procedure because it is exactly that: simple and effective.

In one case, a woman completely stopped her migraine headaches, from which she had suffered for five years. This she did in only three procedures.

In another interesting case, one woman suffered from constant fatigue and muscle pain. Her blood test was seriously abnormal showing life-threatening factors. After eight weeks of doing the Whole Digestive System Cleansing$^{\circ}$ each week, she started feeling a surge of energy which she has not felt in years. The pain in her muscles disappeared, and the primary amazing result was that her blood test became ideal.

Whole Digestive System Cleansing© is also helpful when combined with other cleansing procedures, increasing the effectiveness of each one. All these procedures, preparations, and performances are described in detail in this book.

Do You Really Want to Be Healthy?

Physical, mental, and emotional energy are required to maintain good health, and even more so to regain good health.

Some people have spent 40 to 50 years ruining the condition of their bodies, and then think they can regain original health within a short time or in a few procedures. They are surprised when they learn that regaining health takes time, effort, energy, change of lifestyle, and healthy eating.

Stop for a moment and think this through. If it took decades to accumulate the poisons that are damaging your health, then it will take at least a little time to remove them. No, it won't take years to reverse the self-inflicted poisoning, but it will take time measured in months, maybe up to a year in severe cases.

The only way you can do it quickly is by the horrible path of surgery. Since toxins are often in all tissues down to the cellular level, can surgery even get them? No. It can remove gross contamination like accumulations in the colon, but at what price to your health? Do you really want to be put to sleep and then cut open to remove these poisons?

Often we hear phrases like, "I don't have time to do these cleansings." Here is something for you to consider.

Let's say that it took you an hour to travel to the Center, and hour in the office, and an hour to travel back home (or to your office). That is three hours. Now let's assume, for the sake of discussion, that you did this once a week for a year. That is 156 hours, or less than a week in terms of hours. Now compare that to the extra **years** of life you can expect because you cleansed your body from toxins. "Nuff said?"

A second consideration is to examine your day, starting with the morning and ending with the evening. Carefully think about each thing you do. Does everything you do have such important meaning to you that you cannot live without it? Is there anything as important to you as your health and life? I am sure that most people will find they waste lots of time on meaningless activities.

Examine your money in the same way. Who can say that he never bought things which he used one two times or never at all? Who can say that she bought only things that are necessary and really needed? Carefully look through your accounts and you will see how much you have spent for things that are meaningless or actually harmful. Get rid of these expenditures and invest in your health instead.

Famous author Neal Walsch claims that he has spoken with God. Once he asked God what to do to be healthy and live longer. God reportedly said, "You ask how to live longer but you, yourself, don't want to live longer." Neal affirmed that he really does want to be healthy, and God answered, "If you wanted to be healthy, you would not be smoking. If you wanted to be healthy, you would not eat meat of dead animals and other products which ruin your health."

Like the famous author, you need to evaluate whether really want to be healthy. To help you discover the strength of your determination, we offer you a test. In this test you need to mark, not the answer which you think is right, but the answer for which you are ready, the one you will do. Only then will you know for sure if you're determined to improve your health. Only then will you know which level of success you can reach.

Test to Determine How Strong Is Your Desire to Get Healthy

For each question, check (✓) all answers that apply:

1. In your opinion, what is the reason for your disease?
   - ☐ Genetics
   - ☐ Stress
   - ☐ Accident
   - ☐ Work in dangerous conditions
   - ☐ Other _____
   - ☐ Don't know

2. Whose responsibility is it that you are ill?
   - ☐ Your spouse
   - ☐ Friends or relatives
   - ☐ Your doctor
   - ☐ Your own laziness
   - ☐ Your unhealthy lifestyle and diet
   - ☐ Other _____
   - ☐ You don't know

3. Are you ready not only to do the cleansing procedures but also to invest your efforts and take your responsibility for your health?
   - ☐ Yes
   - ☐ No

4. The following are difficulties which may arise along your way. Which ones are you ready to meet?
   - ☐ Feeling worse before you get better
   - ☐ Staying on a plateau for awhile where nothing changes
   - ☐ Waking up 30 minutes or more earlier to walk and do other exercises
   - ☐ Refusing your favorite food:
     - ☐ Sweets
     - ☐ Meat
     - ☐ Ice Cream
     - ☐ Coffee
     - ☐ Other _____

5. Which of the following bad habits are you ready to quit or stay quit?

Quit	StayQuit	
☐	☐	Smoking
☐	☐	Alcohol
☐	☐	Drugs
☐	☐	Sitting for long periods watching television
☐	☐	Others

_____

6. Are you ready to resist pressure from friends and relatives to break your chosen healthy way?
   - ☐ Yes
   - ☐ No

7. What effort are you ready to put out to get healthy?
   - ☐ A little
   - ☐ Moderate amount
   - ☐ Whatever it takes

8. How much money are you ready to spend to get healthy, that is for cleansing procedures, consultations, books, supplements, kitchen equipment, and health equipment?
   □ $75
   □ $300
   □ $1,000
   □ $10,000
   □ Whatever it takes

9. How much time are you ready to spend to get healthy?
   □ One week
   □ One month
   □ One year
   □ Whatever it takes

10. Which of the following is more important in your life than your health?
   □ Money
   □ Job or work
   □ Car
   □ Other _____
   □ Nothing at all

The natural, internal cleansing techniques offered by our Center have a 100% potential to help you regain your maximum possible health and sustain it. To greatly increase your chances of success, you need to add to our work your conscious desire and efforts. The amount of effort you put together with us to fight your disease is the amount of success you get.

Step #1

Colon Cleansing

"The essential foundation for personal health."

What Is Colon Hydrotherapy?

Colon hydrotherapy is a gentle, natural method of washing *long-term* wastes from the entire colon. When this is done, the body no longer has to deal with wastes accumulated during a lifetime, and can use more of its own strength to heal itself and fight disease.

Who Needs Colon Hydrotherapy?

Virtually everyone has these built-up wastes in the colon. Most people in developed countries eat a lot of processed foods. As these (unnatural) foods move through the colon, fluids are absorbed during the digestive process, and a very sticky waste is created. These wastes cling to the colon walls and rot, releasing toxins that the body has already rejected.

How Does Colon Hydrotherapy Work?

Colon hydrotherapy uses state-of-the-art equipment to gently introduce purified water into the colon. During a colon hydrotherapy session, the pressure and temperature are controlled by a trained and experienced colon hydrotherapist who stays right there with the client. The therapist keeps the temperature and pressure at comfortable levels based on the client's feelings and instructions.

Is Colon Hydrotherapy Safe and Sanitary?

Yes. Each client receives his or her own brand-new speculum and plastic hose, which are immediately disposed of after use. Since all water and wastes are completely contained in a closed system, there is no mess and no odor. The client's dignity is preserved by the use of private draping and room. The procedure is professionally performed and preserves modesty.

Is Colon Hydrotherapy Painful or Dangerous?

No. The pressure is less than that of naturally occurring gas. The most one feels is the urge to have a bowel movement. This urge is satisfied by the work of the constantly circulating water, which removes first the new waste, then the old, long-term wastes.

How Many Colon Hydrotherapy Sessions Does a Person Need?

It took a long time to build up the long-term wastes in your colon, so in order to remove them gently, it will take more than one session. Depending on one's personal health, level of toxicity, and desire to improve, a person might need ten to twelve sessions. After the series, a person might want to cleanse once a month.

Can Colon Hydrotherapy Affect the Flora Balance?

Good flora does not usually predominate in colons that have old wastes stuck to their walls. Colon hydrotherapy washes out, not only the bad flora, but also the environment in which it grows. Then good flora has the opportunity and ability to thrive in a clean environment.

Can Colon Hydrotherapy Affect the Electrolyte Balance?

Colon hydrotherapy has very little effect on the balance of electrolytes. The few that are lost are replaced by proper eating or by the fresh juices that you might drink later.

Can Colon Hydrotherapy Help to Control Weight?

Research from scientists in both America and Europe have demonstrated that people in the richer nations carry within their bodies anywhere from 10 to 50 pounds of accumulated toxic materials. Although this material is stored throughout the body, the majority of it is stored in the colon. Accumulated toxic waste materials slow down metabolism, beginning after age 25 or 30. Colon hydrotherapy helps a person to lose the toxic weight and to increase the metabolic rate at the same time.

Instructions
for
Colon Cleansing

1. Don't eat or drink anything for two hours before the procedure.
2. For best results we suggest you not eat any foods that produce gases, such as beans, cabbage, cauliflower, broccoli, nuts, and bread, on the day the procedure will take place.
3. Avoid soft drinks on the day you'll have the procedure done. (In fact, avoid soft drinks altogether.)
4. For those who suffer from bloating, don't eat any raw fruits, vegetables or beans for 24 hours before and after the procedure. It is better to eat whole grains (brown rice, buckwheat, millet, quinoa, amaranth) steamed vegetables and freshly made vegetable juices.
5. If you have never had a colonic before, or haven't had one for a long time, it is much better if you have a colon cleansing 2 or 3 days in a row; this will help soften and eliminate hard clogs and colon stones, and it will also help eliminate a lot of gases, which may give you bloating and pain. Then you may continue the cleansing once or twice a week. (The recommended number or frequency of procedures given upon individual considerations).

6. If you are too blocked and full with gas, it is normal to feel some discomfort after the procedure. If you experience pain or other problems that bother you, you may drink hot water (1 cup water plus 1 teaspoon lemon juice), 2 sips every 5 minutes, or put a pinch of sea salt under your tongue, until the salt is diluted. Then swallow the saliva and spit out any remaining salt grains. This helps to neutralize toxins, and you will start feeling better. If you need to, you can call us for consultation.

7. If you suffer from chronic hemorrhoids you may expect some discomfort in the rectum and sometimes a little blood. If you have chronic colitis, is possible that you may see some mucus with blood. If you have sluggish colon or suffer from constipation, after the cleansing you probably won't feel the need to have a bowel movement for 2 to 3 days. *When the Cleansing Program is completed you'll be rid of all these problems.* For your homework to help with this problem, read my book, *Healing through Cleansing, Book 3.*

8. To maintain a clean colon after you have completed a series of cleansings, it is recommended to go on a prevention program described in a later chapter of this book, entitled, "Maintenance Program."

9. Keep in mind that the toxins from the colon go first to the liver. When the liver becomes blocked they spread to other organs and systems, and clog blood vessels.

10. Keeping your colon clean can help you avoid many health-related problems, and also feel and look better, younger and more energetic.

11. To activate the cleansing cycle, it is recommended to follow a cleansing diet. See my book, *Deep Internal Body Cleansing,* chapter entitled, "Diet for Rational Health."

12. At the same time, in order to soften the toxic waste in the colon, it is a good idea to have a warm bath for 15 to 20 minutes, two to three times a week.

13. If, during the procedure you don't release a large amount of waste material and you feel discomfort, this is a sign that you are too blocked and your colon is weak. In this case, and in addition to the warm bath, you can put some castor oil compresses on the abdominal area. For this, follow the technique of the castor oil pack discussed later.

14. If, after colon cleansing, you feel cramping, it means that the water from the cleansing awakened the colon and activated peristaltic activity. The colon is now trying to push out the poisons which stick to its walls. Feelings of discomfort after the procedure mean that the muscle movements meet the resistance of blockages, hard and large masses which block the passages. The muscles are not able to overcome the resistance and break up the blockage, so they increase their tension, and this makes you feel cramping. As feces gathers and expands the space behind the blockage, you may feel some pain. Another possible reason for post-cleansing cramping is that one part of either the large or small intestine may be crossed over and constricting another part. To help the colon to break up the blockages and eliminate the mass of gas, it is necessary to do cleansing 2-3 or more days in a row, do abdominal massage, use the castor oil pack, take a warm bath, and drink a lot of liquid.

15. **To open more cleansing channels,** you can combine colon cleansing with FIR (cleansing from heavy metals), IOM (internal organ massage), infrared sauna, and full body cleansing massage.

Castor Oil Pack

1. Buy castor oil from a drug or grocery store.
2. Warm 4-8 oz. castor oil in a small jar or pan.
3. Cut a piece of sheet to size to cover the abdominal area all the way around to the sides.
4. Soak the piece of sheet in the warm oil and then spread the sheet over the abdomen.
5. Cover the sheet with plastic, maybe from a plastic bag.
6. Cover the plastic with a towel.
7. Apply moderate heat by hot water bottle or heating pad next to the towel.
8. Keep this castor oil pack in place for two hours.
9. Shower to clean the oil off.

It is better to do this castor oil pack on the day before Colon Cleansing.

Colon Cleansing is the basis of all cleansings and is included in other cleansing procedures, such as cleansing for kidneys, joints, parasites, and others.
Colon Cleansing relieves pressure in the abdominal area and creates a condition which works like a magnet for toxic biles, toxic mucous, crystals, stones, parasites and other toxic waste. All these poisons are drawn into the colon and then expelled.

Some Disorders and Illnesses Which Could Be Solved with Colon Cleansing

Constipation, gas, bloating, yeast infection, tiredness, skin problems, parasites, bad breathing, abdominal pain, depression, ...

Step #2

Small Intestine Cleansing

"Establishing healthy flora for normal digestion."

The Small Intestine as the "Abdominal Brain"

The small intestine is that part of the digestive tract between the stomach and the large intestine. It is one of the largest organs in the human body, and in adults can be as long as 30 feet. Together with the colon, it makes up the abdominal cavity.

The small intestine takes over where the stomach left off, further digesting the food eaten. Bile is mixed with the partially digested food to increase the effect of pancreatic juices that break down fats.

Although children may refer to this area of the body as the "tummy," in the East it is referred to as the "abdominal brain." This is because this intriguing organ not only digests food, but it also "digests" emotions.

The many different negative emotions are stored in very different but specific parts of the small intestine in the form of constrictions and curves. For example, anger tightens the right part of the small intestine near the liver. Nervousness affects the upper left part of the small intestine under the spleen.

Impatience and anxiety affect the middle of the upper portion of the small intestine, while sadness attacks both sides of the lower parts. Fear, as may be expected, reaches into the deep lower parts.

On a physical level alone, the small intestine is vulnerable to another concern, and that is the long-term accumulation of wastes that build up due to incomplete digestion. These wastes line the small intestine and basically form a toxic layer that releases toxic chemicals into the bloodstream. These slowly acquired wastes also form an optimal environment for parasites to grow.

When the small intestine is overloaded with such toxins, it slows down the digestive process, and decreases its absorbing function. In this situation a person can eat large amounts of food and still be undernourished.

If the small intestine is overloaded with toxins, it loses its natural *tone* and begins to expand. (In fact, some of the large "bellies" you can see are a result of this.) This now larger and heavier organ puts pressure on other, underlying organs in the abdominal cavity and harms their health. Pressure on the veins interferes with circulation and can lead to varicose veins and hemorrhoids. In women, it can lead to menstrual disorders.

The extra weight of the unhealthy small intestine can even begin to pull on the spine, causing various back problems. This in turn can affect the diaphragm and cause imperceptible breathing difficulties.

An unhealthy small intestine increases the production of mucous in the lungs making sinus conditions more troublesome. Even the lymphatic system is impacted by an unclean small intestine.

Combine a physically unclean small intestine with long-term stored negative emotions and one sets the stage for bad health. This is why it is so very important to have a healthy small intestine. The best way to achieve this to practice a proper diet combined with **cleansing** this important organ of long-term wastes that have accumulated over a lifetime.

At the Center for Health and Rejuvenation we have a natural, gentle method of cleansing the small intestine. Based on centuries-proven techniques, the Center can help the body discharge this unwanted waste so that digestion will be improved, and so that the body will not have to spend precious energy fighting the toxins that come from this waste. Overall health will be improved by a strengthened immune system. This will help with the release of the negative emotions that are also stored in this vital organ.

Instructions
for
Small Intestine
Cleansing

Cleansing from Parasites, Yeast, and Heavy Metals

During the Whole Digestive System Cleansing© in our Center, we partly cleanse the small intestine from toxicity; however, the walls of the small intestine are still covered with a thick layer of sticky toxic mucus wherein reside many unfriendly bacteria and parasites.

Because the small intestine carries many nutrients, it attracts many parasites, bacteria, and yeasts to reside there. Parasites which live in the small intestine try to stay closer to the walls in order to steal more nutrients through contact with the blood, and in order to avoid being ejected. Toxic mucus not only sticks to the walls of the small intestine but also seeps inside those walls.

Next, on the walls of the small intestine there accumulate a lot of toxic bile and poisonous heavy metals. Because the small intestine is an organ of absorption, part of these metals' poisons absorb into the blood and lymph, going to the liver, glands, and even the brain. When toxic metals reach the brain, they destroy brain circulation and can cause memory loss and foggy thinking and many other problems.

To flush out this sticky mucus; and eliminate all parasites, yeast, and poisonous heavy metals from the small intestine is not so easy. The only procedure able to do that effectively is the Small Intestine Cleansing© which was created in our Center. After the first procedure, with clean walls of the small intestine, the solution you drink will work like a magnet and will pull toxins and heavy metals from the blood vessels and lymph through the wall of the small intestine and will flush it through the same channel, the small intestine and the colon.

To get the best results from this procedure, it is necessary to start eating right, to do a Parasite Cleansing, to start taking friendly bacteria orally and by implantation directly through the rectum, repeating Small Intestine Cleansing 2-5 times and in some cases even more.

Preparation

For two to three days before the procedure, follow a vegetarian diet of foods that are rich in fiber: fresh fruits and vegetables, whole grains, dried (and soaked overnight)fruits, nuts and seeds.

Then 24 hours before the procedure, begin juice fasting. This means that the only food you will have is freshly made juices from carrots or other vegetables, water and herbal teas.

For those who have yeast problems, it is better to avoid sweet juices and drink green juices from cucumber, celery, spinach, etc., with 30-40% apple or carrot juice for taste. Grapefruit juice is also acceptable.

During this 24 hours, one should drink 1-2 cups of these fluids approximately every two hours during the day to maintain energy. This will also alleviate hunger. Laxatives and enemas are not recommended.

If you suffer from constipation and your colon doesn't eliminate its waste every day, you must have a colonic three days before the procedure. It would also beneficial to take a warm bath for 15 to 20 minutes one day before the procedure. Please wear loose-fitting clothes that do not constrict your circulation or movement in the large intestine. The loose clothing is also appropriate since you will be doing some **mild** exercises.

Performing the Procedure

The cleansing of the small intestine can be done only on an empty stomach.

Performing the procedure includes:
- Drinking a natural, organic solution (liquid) that is prepared and provided by the Center.
- Performing some very mild "exercises" under the direction of Center personnel trained in this procedure.
- Receiving a special abdominal massage. This massage opens the valves in the digestive tract and helps the solution to move more quickly and effectively through the small intestine.
- Drinking some of the solution again.
- Doing the mild "exercises" again.
- Receiving the massage again.
- At this point, most people feel the urge to go to the bathroom. This is where the cleansing is realized.
- This cycle is repeated as needed.

The above procedure will stimulate the entire digestive tract to eliminate waste. At first you will eliminate regular feces. Then the elimination will become more watery. **Our**

**goal is to expel liquid with the same color and
consistency as the solution you have been drinking.**

After the procedure you will receive a meal of carefully
cooked brown rice (or other whole grain) without salt or
other spices. We add only Ghee (clarified butter) to this.
You are allowed to eat only 7-9 ounces of rice or less, even
if you are still hungry. You need to chew your meal slowly
and properly, trying to chew every mouthful 50 to 100
times. **If you are using this procedure to begin a fast, you
will not receive this meal.**

After Your First Meal

One or two hours after your first meal you may drink
spring or distilled water. You may also drink chamomile or
mint tea, with no sweeteners.

For lunch you may choose another grain meal, with
well-steamed vegetables (carrots, onions, celery, etc.) and
Ghee or cold pressed olive oil. In this meal you may add, if
you want to, a little sea salt.

**Do not eat raw vegetables or fruits, dairy products,
meat, or spices**. On the first day, even if you are a raw
foodist, it is better not to eat any raw vegetables or fruits. **It
is necessary to strictly follow this eating program for at
least one day!**

Diet for the Days Following the Cleansing of the Small Intestine

On the next day, you may go back to your regular diet.
For those who have been suffering from bloating, or if you
have candida or other digestive problems, it is important to

establish the a healthy environment in the digestive tract. This includes proper conditions for the development of friendly bacteria whose natural job is to promote good digestion.

With this goal in mind:

1. Eat cooked vegetarian food for 3-5 days.
2. Follow the proper food combining rules. (Provided by the Center.)
3. Take acidophilus orally and through the rectum with a special syringe.
4. Don't eat sweets, or even honey.
5. After the period of eating only cooked vegetarian food, then eat lots of garlic and onions for at least 3-5 days.
6. Properly chew your food. This will help you release lots of saliva, which has disinfectant and cleansing properties.

Suggestions and Explanation for the Cleansing of the Small Intestine

1. Sip the solution. Do not rush, and don't drink too slowly. The drinking speed for one cup is approximately 1-3 minutes.
2. On the day of the small intestine cleansing you will likely feel tired and but relaxed. This is normal because you are spending lots of energy getting rid of poisons and negative energy that was in your digestive system. If you need to, you may rest and sleep after the procedure. Please don't plan too many activities for the rest of the day after this procedure. In fact, you might consider planning to read a book or some other relaxed activity. After the Small Intestine Cleansing, most people feel relaxed and cheerful.

3. ***Before*** the procedure, the digestive system is usually overloaded with food, and creates pressure on the surrounding organs. ***After*** the Small Intestine Cleansing, practically the whole digestive system is completely empty, creating a mild negative pressure. To fill the digestive system again after your have resumed eating normally takes 24-36 hours, perhaps more. **During this time, the negative pressure created by an empty digestive system intensively pulls toxins from the other organs.** (This is actually a change in "toxic pressure" causing toxins to migrate to the area of low toxic pressure, the small intestine.) This means that in 2-5 days after this cleansing, the small intestine will likely accumulate a large amount of toxins. This sudden influx of toxins (not food) creates a noticeable change in this organ. You may begin to feel some discomfort. These toxins will naturally move to the large intestine. Therefore, it is recommended that you do a Colon Cleansing during this time to help the body to get rid of these toxins.

4. The time from your first meal to your first bowel movement is a real transition time for the digestive and elimination systems. If this time is more than 36 hours, it indicates weak digestion and constipation. This is valuable information in that it gives a clearer understanding of an underlying condition in your digestive system. Steps can be taken.

5. To eliminate parasites and their eggs, to get rid of yeast, and to improve digestion, it is recommended to repeat the cleansing of the small intestine four or five times, leaving a break of two or three weeks in between. When you reach your goal, and to maintain this good level, you can repeat this procedure once or twice a year, or more often if your particular situation calls for it.

Re-Colonizing Friendly Bacteria

Small Intestine Cleansing creates optimal conditions for the development of friendly bacteria. First it removes toxins and other negative environmental conditions that make it difficult for friendly bacteria to thrive. Secondly, it creates a healthy environment for the establishment and maintenance of friendly bacteria.

The best re-colonization results occur when the re-colonizing of friendly bacteria comes from two directions, through the mouth and through the rectum. To implant friendly bacteria into the colon, we use a special "syringe" with a two-ounce volume. Be assured that this syringe does NOT have a needle. But it can gently insert the friendly bacteria directly into the colon. From there, the colon knows what to do.

Using a syringe is better than using an enema because using a syringe prevents air from entering the colon. This helps in keeping the solution with friendly bacteria in the colon for a long time. A clean colon creates the best condition for the fast multiplication of friendly bacteria.

Technique to Perform for Re-Colonizing Friendly Bacteria

The procedure is to be performed before you go to bed.

1. In a cup pour 2 oz. clean, purified water.
2. Open 1-2 capsules of friendly bacteria and empty them into the water.
3. Stir.
4. You may also add 1-2 tsp. Of wheat grass juice or chlorophyl.

5. Be sure plunger of syringe is fully depressed to remove all air from syringe.
6. Submerge tip of syringe in solution.
7. Draw plunger back to fill syringe.
8. Lubricate the tip of the syringe with petroleum jelly or preferably with oil.
9. Lie down on your left side and gently insert syringe in rectum.
10. Push in plunger slowly to release the solution.
11. Remove syringe gently, wrap it in a paper towel, and let it remain in a safe place nearby, to be cleaned in the morning.

Repeat this procedure 3-7 days in a row and then 1-2 times per week during 3 or more months.

Therapeutic Effect of the Procedure

- The Small Intestine Cleansing practically cleans your whole digestive system from toxins and parasites.
- The liquid used for the procedure has a high concentration of minerals, and it works like a magnet.
- It pulls toxins from the tissues (which have less concentration of minerals) through the digestive walls and eliminates them with the feces.
- By cleansing tissues in your body you are really cleansing cells.
- This procedure will help to relax tensions and release negative emotions that are also stored in this vital organ.
- Small Intestine Cleansing cleans the digestive buds, which helps to improve the absorption of nutrients and increases digestion.

- Small Intestine Cleansing activates and improves the function of the pancreas and liver, and opens the way for direct cleansing of these vital organs.
- If you suffer from constipation, 3-5 Small Intestine Cleansings will help you overcome this problem.
- A series of these cleansings will dramatically increase your energy.
- Together with Colon Cleansings, the Small Intestine Cleansing improves the form or shape of your abdomen This because a colon and small intestine which are packed full of feces will push out your abdomen to look enlarged and unattractive.
- After the cleansing of both your colon and your small intestine, your abdomen will have a more attractive appearance and give you a thinner look.

Some Disorders and Illnesses Which Could Be Solved with Small Intestine Cleansing

Indigestion, gas, bloating, parasites, constipation, negative emotions, skin disorders, chronic fatigue, sinus problems, pancreas disorders, diabetes, ...

Step #3

Stomach Cleansing

"Removes the damage caused
by years of bad eating."

The Importance of Stomach Cleansing to Your Health

The stomach is that very important organ where either good health or bad health begins.

This is true because the stomach begins the digestive process where your food is separated into nutrients your body needs and waste materials that carry toxins.

Over time, the waste that is not properly removed from the body will stick to the walls of the digestive tract. These wastes build up, thin layer upon thin layer just like plaque in the arteries. Gradually, these layers thicken and create a perfect environment in which disease bacteria, parasites and other unhealthy micro-organisms can thrive.

If this waste lining is not periodically removed it will also interfere with the *production* of digestive juices, and the proper *mixing* of these gastric juices with the chyme.

Poor eating habits are to blame for a variety of stomach problems. Some of those poor eating habits include the following:

1. *Overeating* causes food to ferment in the stomach.
2. *Improper food combinations* cause incomplete digestion, thereby creating excess waste.
3. *Eating "fast foods"* introduces chemical additives which poison the body.
4. *Eating before going to sleep* stresses the entire digestive system. Your body is supposed to be at rest, yet because of food in the stomach, it has to work during sleep. Digestion takes a lot of energy.

As a result of these unfortunate conditions, the body wastes precious disease-fighting energy in inefficient, poorly timed digestion, and on fighting the unwelcome micro-organisms that grow in the uncleansed digestive tract. This can lead to symptoms ranging from acid indigestion and acid reflux, to constipation, gastritis, and ulcers, plus diseases such as cancer.

There are 24,000 new cases of stomach cancer in the United States each year. Although the cause for stomach cancer is not certain, there is an association with gastritis.

One cause of ulcers and gastritis are infections from the recently discovered bacterium *Heliobacter pylori*. Such micro-organisms cannot live in clean, healthy stomachs. Therefore, it is essential that the stomach be kept cleansed to keep this and other bacteria from growing.

Critical to your personal health is the fact that the stomach provides nutrients to the different organs of the immune system. It also supports the good bacteria that inhabit the colon, and controls the proper elimination of wastes. Therefore, good nutrition combined with cleansing the digestive system are vital to developing and then preserving good health.

In order to remove these problems, regular cleansing of the stomach is needed. Stomach Cleansing uses natural methods, gently and safely, to cause the stomach to release these long-term, accumulated wastes for elimination. This procedure removes the environment required by parasites and harmful micro-organisms. With these unwelcome life forms gone, the immune system no longer needs to fight them.

By removing stored wastes, Stomach Cleansing removes poisonous chemicals and harmful bacteria (toxins) that are an additional burden to the immune system. This permits the immune system to fight diseases and invading bacteria with greater strength and effectiveness.

Stomach Cleansing is one technique used as part of the program of "Deep Internal Body Cleansing." Using herbs, organic juices and massage, "Deep Internal Body Cleansing" can cause the body to release wastes that poison the immune system and interfere with its ability to heal itself.

This procedure can only be properly accomplished by trained, experienced professionals who understand these techniques. The Center for Health and Rejuvenation has more than a half century of professional experience in "Deep Internal Body Cleansing" techniques that help the body flush away wastes and heal itself. The Center has both up-to-date equipment and international experience that together provide the maximum in internal cleansing.

Instructions
for
Stomach Cleansing

"Cleansing the upper stomach through regurgitation or vomiting."

Benefits

- Enhances your digestion.
- Activates the function of the pancreatic glands and liver.
- Cleanses the stomach from stagnated bile.
- Purges mucus from the bronchus and lungs.
- Helps lessen the symptoms of allergies, nasal congestion, colds, flu, etc.
- Expels poisonous matter from the stomach through a powerful technique.
- Improves mood, emotions, and outlook on life.
- Calms the nerves and spirit.

Description of Technique

Materials to have on hand include a tub of several gallon size capacity, paper towels or napkins, and a wet face cloth.

1. Cleansing of the upper stomach (that bulbous part that first receives food) must be done only on an empty stomach, and preferably in the morning after toiletries and morning exercises. (If necessary, this procedure can be done at any time as long as the stomach is empty.)

2. First drink two or three glasses of the solution provided. Drink it in the kitchen or in the restroom while either sitting or squatting comfortably. Make sure your spine is straight while drinking the solution. Sit in a straight-backed chair or stand or walk. If you bend forward while drinking you squeeze the stomach. The speed of drinking should be rather fast, a cup every 1-2 minutes, in order to lessen absorption. (The virtue of this solution is not in being absorbed as if it were food.)

3. Throughout the procedure, do the steps calmly and deliberately. It is important not to strain or stretch your muscles.
   - Wash your hands thoroughly
   - Position yourself near the tub.
   - Wet two fingers in clean warm water but do not wipe them dry. Leave them wet.
   - Close your eyes, and put the other hand on your stomach. Make a fist with that other hand and press inward and upward on the upper abdomen to help the stomach release its contents.
   - Take a deep, slow breath.

- Put the two wet fingers down your throat and press down on the root of the tongue to stimulate the "gag reflex."
- Bend slightly over the tub, exhale, and then vomit a small amount in one or two cycles. **Do this gently.**
- **Note:** This is not the same as nausea. This is a highly controlled activity or movement. It is done from the mind, and with the same precision as an exercise. Think in terms of simply emptying the contents of the stomach. Because your stomach is empty except for the solution, the sensation will not be anywhere near as unpleasant as vomiting partially digested food.

Caution: Don't try to empty the stomach 100% because that can stress the heart or cause you to feel discomfort and tiredness.

- Take long, deep breaths through your mouth by inhaling gently along the two fingers still inserted in your mouth. (Be careful not to gulp or gasp air.) Deep, slow breathing is important.
- After one vomiting cycle, clean your fingers, mouth, face, and nose with running water under the faucet, with a paper towel, or with a cool, wet face cloth previously placed within reach.

4. Drink two or three more glasses of solution.

5. Repeat again one or two cycles of vomiting.

6. Drink two to four more glasses of solution.

7. Try to vomit with more strength and volume, while being careful not to stress yourself too much.

8. Take a 30 to 60 second break between cycles.

   "Divided Drinking" is a technique of drinking the warm water solution in stages, not all at once. This technique is beneficial because with every repeated cycle of "divided drinking," the vomiting becomes easier. This is a benefit not found by drinking the solution all at once and regurgitating it all at once. Another benefit of "divided drinking" is that by not filling the stomach to the limit, you prevent that over-full feeling, and you do not stress the heart.

9. The final period of cleansing comes when all of the solution has been drunk. **This period is very important.** During this time, without drinking, try to empty the stomach as much as possible, making the rest of the solution come up. Divide this final period into cycles, taking breaks between cycles. Breaks should last 30 seconds in the beginning, then increase to one minute then to three minutes and more. This gives you more rest, and a better opportunity to listen to your body to find the best moment to vomit. Continue to vomit until you sense the bitter taste, see the yellow color of bile, and feel the burping stop. Finish when you feel calm and empty inside.

10. To bring your stomach to a balanced, normal condition in which it feels calm and relaxed, drink one-half glass of cool, pure water, or an herbal tea. This tea can be made from camomile, but without honey. Then take a warm shower, lie down, and relax. Even though the entire procedure must take about one hour, the active cleansing will take 20 to 30 minutes.

11. Do not eat anything for a minimum of three hours after completing this procedure. Let this organ rest.

12. If you are experiencing any stomach problems, eat well-cooked brown rice or buckwheat with butter, but no sooner than three hours after the procedure. This tends to settle the stomach.

13. If you are not having stomach problems, (usually the case) you may eat vegetarian meals.

14. It is better to learn this procedure under professional supervision. After you become proficient in it yourself, you should consider repeating this procedure about every two to four weeks for maintenance purposes.

15. If you do not practice good eating habits, and/or if you have a candida overgrowth, it may be necessary to do this procedure more often.

Signs of Candida Overgrowth

1. The urine is not clear, possibly with bubbles and foam.
2. Feces float because the gasses produced by candida are mixed with the feces.
3. Discomfort in the stomach, or in the abdomen area (excessive burping, bloating, gas, etc.).

(You can find other symptoms in Donna Gates' book, *The Body Ecology Diet*.)

How to Make the Solution

Take 1-3 quarts of clean purified water, and warm it to body temperature. (Do not use a microwave oven for this.) Add 1 teaspoon of sea salt per 1 quart of water and mix thoroughly.

Caution

Don't do this procedure if you have high blood pressure or a serious heart problem. In this case, do an easier variation of Stomach Cleansing which is described in my book, *Healing Through Cleansing*, Book 3. Also use this alternative technique if you don't have a natural gag reflex.

Some Disorders and Illnesses Which Could Be Solved with Stomach Cleansing

Weak digestion, nausea, headache, sinus problems, burping, sore throat, colds, flu, coughing, asthma, allergies, ...

Step #4

Complex Liver Cleansing

"Helping your major blood filter to normalize cholesterol."

The Liver: Your First Line of Defense Against Disease

The liver is the most important organ in the entire human immune system because its primary function is to remove harmful chemicals and unwelcome microscopic organisms that cause disease.

Sources of chemical and biological toxins are numerous in our environment, and include automobile and truck exhaust, preservatives commonly used in processed foods, nicotine, chemical fumes from manufactured products, airborne dust and microbes, pharmaceuticals and other drugs, alcohol, fats in foods, and poorly cleaned foods. As these toxins enter the human body, they will slowly poison your health unless removed.

The way the liver removes these contaminants is by filtering them from the blood stream, and then sending these poisonous wastes to the excretory organs. As it goes about the business of filtering, the liver too often experiences the very same problem all filters have: It becomes clogged with the material which it is filtering. This leads to three problems.

First, the contaminants clogging the liver are literally stored in this organ instead of being transported for removal via urination or defecation. As these unwelcome chemicals and microscopic organisms accumulate and concentrate over time, the liver is slowly poisoned by them.

Second, toxins stored in the liver build up in size over time and create very real physical pressure inside the liver. This physical pressure interferes with the ability of fluids to flow freely within the liver. It impairs the blood's access to the filtering work of the liver.

Third, because these contaminants clog the liver, its ability to filter out new contaminants is lessened. The amount of this decrease in function is proportional to the amount of filter pores which are clogged. Since the liver is not able to filter at maximum efficiency, toxins are not being removed from the blood stream. This means more chemical and biological toxins are circulated to all of the organs and tissues in the body. These toxins are stored at the cellular level and slowly poison those organs and tissues.

The bottom line is that a liver bloated with masses of chemical and biological toxins is not only less able to fight simple sicknesses such as colds and flu, but is weakened in the fight against the more serious diseases such as cancer, etc.

Add to this the toxins building up in the rest of your body and you get poor health generally, and an increased vulnerability to the diseases to which you are genetically prone. Since **the liver is the power player in the immune system**, you cannot afford to have your star athlete in the game of good health to be on the bench or on the way to the hospital because modern contaminants have begun to choke the life out of it.

The famous Indian doctor Shevananda said that about 90% of health disorders come from a weakened liver. The latest medical research shows that all degenerative diseases (cancer, arthritis, diabetes, asthma, etc.) are created by the dysfunction of a liver which is blocked and overloaded with toxic waste material.

Side Effects of Having a Toxic Liver

The liver performs other critical functions. It participates in digestion, metabolism, and the proper working of the gall bladder.

The gall bladder and the liver work in close harmony as well as close proximity. Accumulated toxins in the liver slow down the secretion of bile from the gall bladder. This results in bile crystallization and the formation of gall bladder stones.

Although the liver is the key organ in the immune system, the lymphatic system, the circulatory system, the spleen, and the bone marrow are also part of the immune system. The stronger each individual member of the immune system is, the better they work together and the stronger the entire immune system is.

An unclean liver means unclean blood which blocks the tiny ducts in the thyroid gland.

The Good News

Fortunately, the health-robbing toxic wastes stored in the liver can be removed naturally under the guidance of a trained professional. Using techniques developed and enhanced over the centuries, the human liver can be coaxed into gently releasing, not only the original contaminants entering the body, but also their by-products such as cholesterol, fat, pathologic mucous, stagnated bile, and bilirubin stones.

Since "an ounce of prevention is worth a pound of cure," a liver cleansing will allow you to take powerful steps towards fighting off life-threatening disease, debilitating illnesses, and common sicknesses. It will help you to feel healthier and enjoy life more since the nasty toxins that once choked your liver are gone.

Nine-Organ Cleansing Procedure

Liver cleansing in our Center is a complex cleansing of nine important body organs: **stomach, pancreas, liver, gall bladder, spleen, small intestine, colon, blood, and thyroid gland.**

Benefits of a Full Complex Liver Cleansing

- Enhanced ability to clean the bloodstream.
- Stronger immune system.
- Loss of toxic waste and weight.
- Improved metabolism.
- Cleaner skin.
- Improved digestion.

- Greater protection from degenerative diseases such as cancer, arthritis, diabetes, and asthma.

Side Benefits of a Liver Cleansing

A full Complex Liver Cleansing automatically cleanses the gall bladder, the pancreatic gland, and the spleen. It also helps cleanse the small intestine and the colon while strengthening the lymphatic and circulatory systems. Additionally, proper liver cleansing improves the tone of the kidneys and the thyroid gland. Clean blood helps to cleanse the thyroid gland and improve its function.

Because the liver is naturally divided into four parts, or quadrants, and since each cleansing will cleanse only one part, **full Complex Liver Cleansing requires four separate procedures.**

During Complex Liver Cleansing, toxic wastes released by the above organs go first into the small intestine then on to the colon. These wastes are then best removed by Colon Cleansing that gently flushes these toxic wastes out of the body before they can adhere to the colon walls.

Instructions
for Complex
Liver Cleansing

Our Complex Liver Cleansing is different from liver cleansings described in other books.

The first disadvantage of other liver cleansings is that you do not have a fully trained health professional—with experience in liver cleansing—to personally tailor the procedure to your particular circumstances.

Second, you have no professional guidance during the procedure, or anyone of whom to ask questions as they arise.

The third disadvantage is the lack of preparation. When one properly prepares for this (or any) cleansing procedure, the procedure is more effective. This is often because the toxic masses and stones (gall stones and liver stones) are softened by proper preparation, and therefore exit more fully from the organ being cleansed. Without this preparation the results are decreased.

The fourth disadvantage is that most liver cleansings do not call for the small intestine to be cleansed prior to the liver cleansing. This is important because the small intestine is the organ into which the liver discards its toxins during the liver cleansing. If the small intestine is blocked with accumulated wastes, the movement of the newly released liver toxins is slowed. When these wastes are slowed down

51

in the small intestine and the colon there is a greater chance for them to stick to the walls of these two organs, and a greater chance that the wastes will be reabsorbed.

Procedures that Prepare the Body for Complex Liver Cleansing

In our Center, we do much preparation before Complex Liver Cleansing. We carefully cleanse the whole digestive system to assist in the removal of toxic bile and other liver wastes (as described above). In addition, we use juice therapy, Far Infrared Radiation (FIR), massage of internal organs, reflexology, and infrared sauna to soften accumulated wastes.

Complex Liver Cleansing is the best beginning for Cell Cleansing. The combination of these two cleansings is a powerful way to help to heal many diseases, rejuvenate the body, and lose toxic weight.

ATTENTION: *Read and understand this material very carefully.*

Preparation for Complex Liver Cleansing

1. *Do a Series of Colon Cleansings and 1-2 Small Intestine Cleansings before the Complex Liver Cleansing.* This is necessary because accumulated toxic waste materials from the liver go through the small intestines and the colon, as described above.

2. One or two weeks before the Complex Liver Cleansing, start to take a warm bath two or three times a week. Don't stay in the bath more than 15 to 20 minutes. Two to three cups of sea salt or Epsom salt can be added to the bath. A warm bath helps to soften up the toxicity and facilitates its removal.

3. Switch to the vegetarian diet for three to seven days before Complex Liver Cleansing. This gives the liver an opportunity to accumulate strength and energy to expel the toxins.

4. Go on juice therapy (juice fasting) for three days right before Complex Liver Cleansing. During these days you may drink distilled water and juices freshly made if possible. During the first two days, drink carrot, carrot-apple, and apple juices at your own discretion. On the third day it is better to drink apple juice only, or the juice of 4-5 apples plus one lemon. Drink one or two glasses approximately every two hours. If possible, use only organic carrots. When choosing the variety of apple, it is preferable to buy "Granny Smith." Juices absorb into the bloodstream, go through the liver, flush it, and activate the flow of stagnated bile. **If you have yeast in your body,** drink 1 cup juice alternating with 1 cup water to dilute the concentration of sugar. Also, you can drink tea made from the dandelion root.

5. On the third day of juice therapy, you will receive a colon cleansing, FIR, a gall bladder / liver massage, a foot reflexology massage, and infrared sauna. To understand FIR, see my book, *Deep Internal Body Cleansing,* chapter entitled, Heavy Metal Cleansing.

These procedures activate the liver, expand its ducts, and prepare the way for the passage of toxins.

The concluding part of the procedure is performed by the client at home after receiving detailed instructions. (See below.) At this time you will pick up from the Center the solution for Complex Liver Cleansing for consumption at home.

The First Day of Complex Liver Cleansing

The first day of Complex Liver Cleansing is the same as the third day of juice therapy (as described above).

This first day is divided into two parts: (a) procedures performed in the Center, and (b) procedures performed at home. (For procedures performed at the Center see #5 above.)

Once you have completed the procedures to be performed in the Center on this first day you will go home with the carefully prepared, organic solution for oral consumption.

At approximately **7:00 p.m.** begin the procedures described below. (This assumes that you normally keep waking hours that most people keep.) The reason for this timing is that the procedures you will perform at home cause the majority of toxins to exit the liver between 1 and 3 a.m. This is the biorhythmic time when the liver is most active. You should be finished with the procedures below in about four hours.

Sequence of Steps:

Notice: Two hours before drinking Solution #1, do not drink anything, including water.

-Prepare your bed
-Put (warmed) solution near your bed.
-Prepare chopped garlic in a closed container.
-Prepare a piece of lemon on a plate near your bed.
-Prepare a piece of pickle on a plate near your bed.
-Have a timer near your bed.

1. Take a warm bath for 15 to 20 minutes. The bath doesn't have to be very hot, but the hotter you can tolerate it the better. At the end of your bath, and before you stand up, flush your face and forehead with cool water. When you stand up from the bath do so very slowly. These precautions are necessary for people with weak vessels and unstable blood pressure, to avoid dizziness and falling. Be careful!

2. From the bath go directly to the bed. Lie down on your right side (where the liver is) with your head and chest elevated so as to create better drainage. Put a very warm heating pad or water bottle under your right side (on the liver area). **IT IS VERY IMPORTANT THAT YOU NEVER FALL ASLEEP ON A HEATING PAD. YOU CAN GET BURNED IN THIS FASHION.** This is another reason for having a timer next to the bed, just in case you fall asleep on the bed. If the heating pad or water bottle is too hot for you, cover it with a towel. Make sure you feel no tightness or contraction in the liver area.

3. Warm the solution provided by the Center in a double boiler pan to body temperature before going to bath, or have someone warm it for you during your bath. If you have a problem drinking it warm, drink it at room temperature.

After lying down on your right side with a heating pad or water bottle, raise your body on your elbow and . . .

a. Drink solution #1.

You will notice that the solution is a two-phase liquid. It is recommended that you do not to try to mix the solution. It is also recommended that you drink the solution with moderate speed without stopping. After you drink the solution, lie down on the heating pad/hot water bottle on your right side immediately. Rest for 15 minutes.

b. Drink solution #2.

Rest 20 minutes.

c. Drink solution #3.

Rest 20 minutes.

d. Drink solution #4.

Rest 25 minutes.

e. Drink solution #5.

Rest 25 to 30 minutes

f. Drink solution #6. (If you are small, the first time you will receive 5 jars instead of 6. If your weight is more than 200 pounds, on the second Liver Cleanse you may receive more than 6 jars.)

Continue lying on your right side for one more hour after you finish drinking the solution. If lying on the right side becomes difficult, it is permitted periodically (for one or two minutes) to turn on your back.

After one hour, it is okay to lie on your back and on your right side. Try not to lie on the left side or on the abdomen.

Everybody is different. If you find it uncomfortable to lie down, you are allowed to sit in a comfortable chair with the heating pad tied snugly around you. One to one-and-one-half (1-1½) hours after drinking your solution, you may lie in bed on your right side or on your back, and drink the solution while in the sitting position.

The drinking solution contains a large amount of oil so there will be a strong impulse from the liver and gall bladder to push out bile to break down the fat. Because the small intestine is empty with the duct open, and the liver contents are softened by juice, it will be able to push out a large amount of toxins like cholesterol, chemicals, medicines, stones and stagnant bile along with the new bile.

From the small intestine, the toxins go to the large intestine and then to the exit. Sometimes, it is possible to hear "the breathing" of the liver, that is, movement of the stones, mucous, stagnated bile, and other toxins.

Some people, as the result of incorrect and excessive food intake, might have a half-open position of the valve between the stomach and small intestines. In this case, dissolved toxic bile, mucous, and other toxic components of the liver which are dissolved because of the drinking solution, and also some of the solution itself, might come through into the stomach and create nausea. This is not unusual.

During light nausea there are some things you can do to help:

1. Open the container with cut garlic and inhale the vapor from it.

2. Gargle with freshly made lemon juice, or suck a piece of lemon (don't eat it).

3. Put a piece of pickle in the mouth and suck the juice from it. Don't eat the pickle.

4. Press on the point of your face, right under your nose and right over your upper lip. Press it for 10 to 15 seconds. Do not press too hard.

If nausea becomes stronger and the above methods don't help, try to tolerate it for two or three hours after drinking the last jar of solution. During this time try to relax and rest; try not to move, or to move as little as possible.

Then, if the nausea has not gone away, try to induce vomiting by stimulating the root of the tongue with two fingers. Do it several times, until your stomach is empty. If vomiting does not happen, drink 1-2 cups of very warm water and repeat stimulation of the root of the tongue. The water will help and make it easier for you to cleanse your stomach. After that, flush your mouth with cool, clean water.

Although it is preferable to have the wastes from the liver exit via colon hydrotherapy, if the body calls for you to vomit this material it is better to do so. You will thank yourself afterward, because you will feel better.

Lie down, relax, and rest. If possible, ask your relatives to massage your feet. Then put a warm water bottle to your feet.

After vomiting, you may experience a burning sensation in your stomach and in your mouth. It is normal and will go away. It happens because of the toxic bile and other materials from the liver.

Thirty minutes to one hour after vomiting, or four hours after drinking the last jar of solution, you may drink hot herbal tea from camomile and peppermint, with honey, which will decrease or even eliminate any unpleasant tastes.

Regardless of the unpleasantness of vomiting, it does have its positive side. It graphically demonstrates what the liver has had to put up with "for all these years."

Vomiting also helps to clean and activate the pancreatic gland, and to clean the bottom of the stomach from stagnated bile and other toxins. It also helps to improve digestion and improves the work of the valve between the stomach and small intestine.

The Second Day of Complex Liver Cleansing

In the morning, after waking up, take a warm shower and clean your teeth, mouth and tongue. Then drink one glass of water with one teaspoon of apple cider vinegar or lemon juice. Do not eat any food before Stomach or Small Intestine Cleansing. If you plan to do a Colon Cleansing, and if you do not feel nauseous, you may drink carrot or apple juice plus beet juice, 1-2 cups.

Do a few gymnastic exercises and light walking.

If you have bowel movements, pay attention to what comes out. You may observe dark green or light green liver stones up to one-half inch in length. These liver stones can assume a variety of shapes, from football to irregular to amorphous. What you are seeing is toxic mucous, toxic bile, excess cholesterol, the residue of alcoholic beverages, drugs (prescription or other), and various other wastes. Sometimes these wastes have a very unpleasant smell. Just remember that you never have to be afflicted with this toxic waste again. It is gone.

Some people are slower to eject toxins from the liver, and some people's systems are slower to move these toxins through the intestinal tract. In this case, you will see toxins from the liver only during the procedure at the office.

The second day must be your day off from work both in the office and at home. Your body has just expended a lot of energy to get rid of decades of toxins so it is normal for you to feel weak. This weakness will be offset by the strength you will begin to gather from having a rejuvenated liver and other organs. Whatever weakness, nausea, and other unpleasant sensations you may experience will go away quickly.

On the second day of Complex Liver Cleansing, you may receive some of the following cleansing procedures:

1. Stomach Cleansing.
2. Colon Cleansing.
3. Small Intestine Cleansing.
4. Sinus Cleansing.
5. Sauna.
6. Full Body Cleansing Massage.

The most important procedure following a Liver Cleanse is Colon Cleansing. Other procedures add benefits and increase the amount of toxins eliminated from the liver and other organs and prevent re-absorption.

30 minutes to 1 hour after colon hydrotherapy, you may eat cooked brown rice with Ghee.

Some Other Useful Advice

1. Try to follow the instructions to the letter. Any changes must be reconciled. Violating instructions will decrease the benefits of the cleansing or may even harm you.

2. During this cleansing, it is not recommended to take any drugs. If you have to take pharmaceuticals, let us know about them before cleansing.

3. Don't combine Complex Liver Cleansing with a dental appointment or with anesthesia. If you need to see a dentist, do it before Complex Liver Cleansing.

4. Don't get upset if during the Complex Liver Cleansing you don't see any stones. Everything you eliminate during the Complex Liver Cleansing (stones, toxic bile, mucus, etc.) is poison and its elimination improves your health. Sometimes good preparation and juices dilute liver and gall bladder stones and transform them to green black, sticky liquid.

First Week after Complex Liver Cleansing

After the procedure of Complex Liver Cleansing, the liver will stay open and continue ejection of toxins for five to seven days.

Some of these toxins will be collecting in the large intestine, so it is recommended to do another Colon Cleansing in 3-5 days after Complex Liver Cleansing.

During this time, you should not overeat or choose gas producing foods such as beans. Gas expands your stomach and creates pressure on the liver. This stops this process of continuing to eliminate toxins.

During these days, the diet must be vegetarian.

You will be surprised to see the toxins coming out. Your liver will receive relief.

Therapeutic Benefits

Benefits derived from a Complex Liver Cleansing are priceless. These include:
- Strengthened immune system.
- Increased energy level.
- Greater sense of well-being.

You will be able to feel this condition only when your liver is completely clean. For this reason, it is necessary to keep on cleansing it until ejection stops.

In the first year, it is recommended to do five to seven Complex Liver Cleansings. The frequency of the procedure depends on individual tolerance.

Then for liver support, one Complex Liver Cleansing per year is enough.

Some Disorders and Illnesses Which Could Be Solved with Complex Liver Cleansing

Gall stones, high cholesterol, allergies, skin problems, digestive problems, hepatitis, thyroid disorders, constipation, headaches, parasites, anger, insomnia, ...

Step #5

Joint Cleansing

"Removing joint pain and
increasing flexibility."

Cleansing the Joints, Spine and Tissues

The pathway to preventing joint pain, and even to
lessening its painful effects for those who already have joint
pain, is found first in understanding its causes and then in
cleansing the body of those causes.

The Cause of It All

It is no surprise to those who suffer from joint pains,
such as arthritis, that the pointed stabbing sensation in those
aching joints comes from the formation of needle-shaped
crystals. These crystals are created from uric acid, a
substance found in animal proteins. The typical American
eats much more meat than people in other cultures, and
consequently we have a high incidence of arthritis in this
country.

Diet is not the only thing that can lead to the formation of uric acid crystals. Heredity and a lack of physical activity play a part as well. Organs that have never been cleansed can tend to create conditions favorable to uric acid formation.

Despite all of this, the prudent person can use his or her mind to prevent joint pain caused by such dietary contamination. Indeed, if the physical condition of the afflicted joints is not too far advanced, it may be possible to decrease the pain or in some cases even eliminate the pain.

Why and How It Hurts

Most uric acid crystals form in joints, including the spinal column around the disks. These crystals are hard enough to cause actual wear and tear to these bones.

Unfortunately, other things also can cause physical injury to the joints and the spine: being overweight, lifting very heavy items, very sharp injuring movements and direct blows to the joints. An insufficient amount of sinovial fluid, which acts as a lubricant for the joints, can also lead to bone wear and tear.

One of the many disadvantages that comes from uric acid crystals is that they put pressure on veins and energy channels making blood and energy circulation slower. This can cause the limbs to get cold more easily, leading to extra stiffness in the joints.

Bony materials are not the only part of the body to suffer from the formation of uric acid crystals. These unwelcome mineral needles can form in soft tissue as well, such as the upper-back/shoulders zone. When they do, they tend to scratch the tissues. The reason for uric acid crystals being formed in soft tissues is usually poor blood circulation. This, in turn, is sometimes the result of sitting in an uncomfortable position for too long, and by stress. With time, if no corrective measures are taken, discomfort and pain can occur and increase in the area of shoulders and neck.

All of these situations and conditions can add together to bring unremitting pain to some people. The goal of the Center for Health and Rejuvenation is to use natural healing techniques to remove one of the greatest causes of joint and spine pain, the uric acid crystals.

Bringing Relief

Employing natural healing techniques developed over the centuries, and using state-of-the-art equipment, the Center for Health and Rejuvenation dissolves the uric acid crystals, causing them to be washed easily out of the joints, spine and tissues. The liquefied uric acid is then transported by the circulatory system from the joints, spine and tissues to the waste elimination organs of the body. There is no other way to remove this source of pain, not even surgery.

If you have a serious problem with your joints because of the accumulation of uric acid crystals, then this cleansing must be repeated four or five times during the first year. Then, depending on your personal circumstances and your lifestyle and dietary choices, Joint Cleansing can be continued one or two times a year.

Therapeutic Effects of Joint Cleansing

- Removes certain unhealthy chemicals from your body, naturally and gently.
- May lessen or eliminate pain in areas affected by uric acid crystals.

- May prevent the onset of illnesses caused by uric acid.
- May increase the flexibility and range of motion in joints and/or the spine.
- May make everyday movement easier and exercise better or possible.
- May increase the blood flow in joints, spine and tissues.
- May increase mental concentration since pain is no longer distracting you.
- May make you less vulnerable to changes in the weather.
- May increase physical energy

The specific benefits that each person experiences depends on many interrelated factors, including your own personal body chemistry, the extent of uric acid development, and your diet and exercise. One thing is undisputed: The gentle, natural removal of uric acid is beneficial to your health, especially to the joints.

Instructions
for
Joint Cleansing

The Causes

What causes the sharp increases in pain that are sometimes felt by those suffering from uric acid crystals?

1. Physical fatigue.
2. Pollution of the large intestine.
3. Poor kidney function.
4. The common cold.
5. Negative energy coming from humidity inside buildings, extra moisture from long rains, etc.
6. Long time spent in places where natural magnetic lines intersect, exposure to powerful electromagnetic vibrations (proximity to electric plants) and underground anomalies (underground water, accumulated metals, alloys, vacuums).
7. Frequent emotional stresses.
8. Not enough water.
9. Use of alcohol and overuse of salt in food.
10. Parasites.

Now that we have a brief background on what causes joint, spine and tissue pain, how do we go about preventing these unwelcome needle-shaped intruders? And how do we go about lessening the joint pain some people suffer from the accumulation of uric acid crystals?

The Program

In order to get the greatest good from this program of cleansing the body of uric acid crystals, one is well-advised to lay a good foundation. This includes the following recommendations

1. Cleanse the large intestine (colon) from waste, parasites, gas and excessive pressure. This will create a condition which works like a magnet for uric acid after their crystals are dissolved in the joints with herbs. Uric acid will be drawn into the colon and eliminated during the Colon Cleansing.
2. Follow this with both Liver and Lymph Cleansing.
3. Practice a raw vegetarian diet. 15% to 20% cooked food is allowed. Organic food is preferred.
4. Maintain a program of exercises for joints and spine.
5. Engage in special mind exercises for joints daily.
6. Use dry heat (dry sauna).

Detailed Instruction for Joint Cleansing
(Duration of cleansing: 3 weeks.)

Start and maintain a vegetarian diet. If your digestion is normal, your food should be 80-85% raw. Joint cleansing is done with the help of special herbs. Because these herbs wash out, not only toxic crystals, but also minerals that are

68

necessary for basic health, these lost, good minerals must be replaced by drinking three or four glasses of freshly made, organic juices, and liquid minerals like seasilver and noni juice. You may choose from the following combinations:

- Carrots and celery (6:2 ratio)
- Carrots, cucumber and beet (10:3:3 ratio)
- Carrots, celery and parsley (9:5:2 ratio)
- Grapefruit

These juices must be made from fresh, ripe produce. They must *never* come from a can. They must never be processed such as dried, frozen, etc.

Because the body is also losing potassium, it is necessary to eat foods which contain potassium. These include: potatoes, millet, bananas, apples, soaked raisins, dried apricots, and apple cider vinegar.

Add flaxseed oil to salads.

Raw products and juices give the body necessary minerals and vitamins; they also cool it down. To restore the heat balance one must:

1. During the day, drink 4 to 6 cups of hot Chinese cleansing tea (calli tea).
2. Every day between 5 p.m. and 9 p.m., take a hot bath with sea salt (3-4 cups of salt for one bath).
3. Daily dry brush massage for 10 minutes.
4. Every day, 30 minutes of mind joint exercises.
5. Procedures in the Center's office:
   Massage and Sauna, 2 or 3 times per week
   Colon Cleansing, 1 or 2 times per week

Directions for Taking the Herbal Solution

3 days of taking herbs
   7 day break
3 days of taking herbs
   7 day break
7 days of kidney cleansing

The process of dissolving the uric acid crystals and making them move from the joints, spine and tissues happens, not only during the days you take the herbs, but also during the breaks. Therefore, one must follow the program in order to make it work at maximum. The Center for Health and Rejuvenation will provide you with packets from which you will make a special solution to enhance the cleansing. These will be taken during the three days of taking herbs.

Method of Preparing the Herbal Solution

Put one packet in a pan with 12 oz. of clean water. Heat to boiling and then let simmer for five minutes. Put this mixture in a thermos and let it stay for three hours. Then strain the solution and put in your refrigerator.

Next day start drinking one teaspoon every 15 minutes until done (6 or 8 hours).

If you miss your planned time to drink, continue with the same amount and scheduled time. Do not increase the dosage as that can be bad for your stomach.

How Does the Elimination of Toxic Crystals Occur?

Elements contained in the herbal solution and the freshly-made juices dissolve the uric acid crystals causing them to wash out easily from the joints, spine and tissues. The dissolved uric acid is then transported by the circulatory system to the kidneys and eliminated with the urine.

For those who want proof that the procedure is working, try the following experiment: Each morning collect your first urine in a clean glass jar. Then leave this urine in a cool, dark place such as a closet that is rarely opened. (Make sure children and pets will not find this collection.) After about three or four weeks kept tightly sealed in a cool, dark place, the uric acid will re-crystalize in the collected urine and precipitate to the bottom of the container. Now you can see what was in your joints, spine and tissues.

Dissolved toxins also flow to the large intestine (colon) during this procedure. This is due to the creation of a lower pressure in the colon as compared to other organs. To help this process, it is recommended that you not eat for four hours after Colon Cleansing. During that time you may drink cleansing tea and freshly-made organic juices. The next Colon Cleansing will show you again how much uric acid can be drawn from your system. You will see this in the color of the wastes.

The hot bath with sea salt and the dry sauna help relieve the load on your kidneys by pulling the toxins through the skin. The dry brush massage activates skin respiration and facilitates the work of the lungs to eliminate toxic gasses formed during the process of cleansing. A long walk of one or more hours activates the lungs and the elimination of toxic gasses.

Mind exercises for joints, not only activate blood flow in the joints and the spine, but also improve the flow of energy through the energy channels and the connection between the brain and the joints.

Directions for Mind Exercises for the Joints

1. Sit in a comfortable chair and close your eyes.
2. Visualize someone standing in front of you at a distance at which you can see that person clearly.
3. Who you choose to visualize is up to you. It should be someone who will not distract you from this mind exercise.
4. Visualize this person doing joint exercises beginning with toes and working all the way to the top of the head, 10 repetitions for each movement.
5. See this person lift the left leg, and curl and relax the left toes ten times.
6. See this person flex the ankle, forward and back, side to side, circular clockwise and then counterclockwise.
7. See this person stretch and bend the knee forward and back, side to side, and circular both directions.
8. See this person move the leg at the hip, forward and back, side to side, and circular both directions.
9. Then see this person do the same with the other leg, toes, ankle, knee, and hip.
10. See this person flex and twist the spine forward and back, sideways, and circular both ways.
11. See this person flex the fingers, wrists, elbows, and shoulders in the same manner, both hands together.
12. See this person turn their neck in all positions and directions.
13. See this person flex the jaw, wiggle the ears, and cut the eyes all around.

Visualizing in this way activates the centers in the brain which are responsible for joint movement. Your visualization of someone else activates your own center. It improves the action of the brain center itself and improves connection between the brain and the joints. The joints become more flexible. It is recommended to do mind exercises for the joints once a day for 10-30 minutes.

Important Note: During joint cleansing, you may experience a "healing event." This is a sensation of general discomfort or pain in some parts of the body due to the dissolved uric acid entering your system. These discomforts are typical and actually natural when you think about the process of cleansing. The discomfort does not last long, and constitutes proof that the cleansing is on-going. If there are places in your body that especially bother you, apply compresses made from five- to seven-day-old urine for two or three hours.

Some Disorders and Illnesses Which Could Be Solved with Joint Cleansing

Joint pain, back pain, arthritis, stiffness in joints, insomnia, ...

Step #6

Kidney Cleansing

"Helping your heart and your sexuality."

Kidney Cleansing to Improve Health and to Live Longer

The kidneys are important to your health because this pair of organs filters harmful wastes from the fluids circulating in your body, and sends these wastes to the bladder for elimination.

If the kidneys are not working properly, wastes remain in the body and poison it. The immune system has to work that much harder to fight these unwanted chemicals. Once these dangerous chemicals are flushed from your body, they cannot continue to stress your immune system.

The kidneys also regulate the level of minerals in the body and your acid-alkaline balance. When we do not drink enough water or fresh, raw juices, our fluid levels fall too low. Minerals build up in the kidneys and kidney stones can form. The kidneys, overworked from mineral deposits, become less efficient and effective. Dysfunction of the kidneys is often the reason for pain in the lower part of the back.

Experts have estimated that a minimum of 3,300,000 Americans do not realize that they have kidney disease. More than 20 million Americans suffer from kidney disease and urinary tract disease while some 80,000 will die of these two diseases in this country this year. It is estimated that 400,000 Americans have kidney stones. And kidney disease does not respect any age group.

Therefore, it is very wise to cleanse the kidneys from the wastes and minerals that have accumulated during a lifetime of eating processed food and food additives (unnatural chemicals) and inhaling various chemicals in our environment. Fortunately, this can be done in a safe and gentle manner using only natural techniques and foods.

Benefits of Kidney Cleansing

- Cleansing the blood, lymph system, ureters, and pancreatic gland plus both kidneys.
- Flushing away "sand," non-organic salt, mucous, kidney stones, and retained fluids.
- Increase the health and functioning of these organs and systems, plus the heart and other organs.
- Toxic weight, swelling in the legs, joint pain, and spine pain might disappear.
- Flexibility will be increased.
- Greater sexual satisfaction, since sexual energy comes from the kidneys.

Kidney Cleansing is usually done after Colon Cleansing. The best result will come if done after Colon Cleansing and Complex Liver Cleansing. The service includes a special diet, special massages, fresh organic juices and herbs, warm baths, and sauna. Depending on the kidney condition and the chosen method, this cleansing can be done over time from one week to one month.

Instructions
for
Kidney Cleansing

For those who are doing Kidney Cleansing as a preventative measure, in order to eliminate sand, small non-organic mineral salt crystals, and mucus, the program will require seven to ten days.

For those who have kidney stones, it may be necessary to repeat this program two or three times, depending on the size and number of these stones. In order to cleanse the kidneys from stones, non-organic mineral salt crystals and mucus, the following conditions must be met:

1. First decrease, and then maintain, a low level of pressure from fecal matter and gases in the abdominal area. High pressure in this area pushes down on the urethra, kidneys and other organs, inhibiting their function and cleansing. This decrease in pressure can be achieved by colon hydrotherapy, and by fasting or eating only small amounts of easily digestible food.

2. Drink a large amount of liquids, such as special juices and herbal extracts. These liquids are capable of dissolving stones and diluting mucous, washing them out of the kidneys.

3. In order to dislodge stones from where they are lodged, it is necessary to perform exercises such as walking, and jumping on a miniature trampoline.

4. To improve the movement of stones through the urethra, the insides of its channels have to be lubricated. Foods which contain lubricant are flax seed and Ghee (clarified butter). Additionally, warm, natural oils rubbed on during a therapeutic massage, can serve as lubricants.

5. During Kidney Cleansing, the workload of the kidney is greatly increased. Whole body massages, reflexotherapy and kidneys massages help the kidneys handle their workload during that time. Also, the Cleansing Sauna, which helps eliminate toxins through the skin, takes a large amount of pressure off the kidneys.

6. It is very important that all channels of the urinary system can be easily widened in order to let big stones through. To achieve this, the body needs to be warmed both internally and externally. This is done by daily warm baths with salts and herbs, and also by drinking hot herbal extracts.

7. Certain Yoga exercises help to activate blood circulation through the kidneys, making them stronger and improving cleansing. These exercises include "The Locust," "The Bow," and "The Cobra." If you are not familiar with these exercises, you may read about them in a book of yoga.

Sample Daily Schedule During Kidney Cleansing

1. After getting up, take a warm shower. Instead of using the towel, dry yourself by using your hands to rub the water off for about 5 minutes.

2. Massage yourself with a dry brush for approximately 5 minutes.

3. Drink one cup of hot Cali tea with half a teaspoon of Ghee.

4. Put your clothes on and do a few yoga exercises to activate kidneys.

5. If you have time take a 30 to 60 minute walk. Dress warmly if it's cold or windy.

6. If you have a trampoline jump for 5 to10 minutes.

7. Before 12 or 1 p.m., you should consume 3 or 4 glasses of juice in the following proportions:
    Carrots -   10 oz.
    Cucumbers - 3 oz.
    Beats -   3 oz.

8. From 12 to 5 p.m., eat watermelon or drink watermelon juice as much as desired.

9. For those who do not wish to lose weight, it is permitted to have a light dinner at 5 or 6 p.m. The amount of food should not exceed 6 to 8 oz. Alternatives for dinner:
   a. Fresh salad of carrots, cucumber, lettuce, celery and lemon juice.
   b. Vegetable soup.
   c. Variety of steamed vegetables.

10. One or one-and-one-half hours after dinner, drink hot Cali tea, with juice from ½ lemon. Stop drinking one hour before going to bed.

11. Every day, for 15-30 minutes, take a warm bath with sea salt, between 5 p.m. and 9 p.m.

12. To create internal lubrication:
    a. Drink hot tea with ½ to 1 tsp. Ghee dissolved in it, 1 or 2 times a day.
    b. Mix 1 glass of water with 1 tsp. flaxseed, heat to boiling, let stand for 10 minutes, and strain. Drink ½ glass twice a day, diluting with water.

13. During Kidney Cleansing, the following procedures are recommended: **Full Body Massage, Colon Cleansing, and Cleansing Sauna.** The frequency of these procedures depends on the individual needs and problems of the patient.

14. If there are kidney stones, special equipment called FIR is used to activate cellular blood circulation and to facilitate the elimination of stones. This procedure also helps in removing heavy metals from the body through the kidneys.

Some Disorders and Illnesses Which could Be Solved with Kidney Cleansing

Water retention, swollen joints, kidney stones, prostate problems, sexual problems, heart problems, lower back pain, heavy metal poisoning, ...

Step #7

Lymph Cleansing

"Increasing the strength of
your immune system."

What Is the Lymph System?

When you eat food, your body digests that food for its
nutrients, and then sends those nutrients to every living cell
in your body. As the cells consume these nutrients some
waste is created. The waste from each cell must be removed
or the body will "drown" in its own waste. The lymph
system, located throughout your body, provides the
"highway" by which this waste is transported from the cells
to the blood to the colon and kidneys. The lymph system
acts as a miniature sewer system.

Why Does the Lymph System Need Cleansing?

The lymph system is more than a transportation system
composed of lymphatic fluids. It also works as a filter,
removing bacteria, microorganisms, dead cells, and other
unwanted substances. Unfortunately, our bodies have an

abundance of these unwelcome substances which can block the lymph nodes, decreasing the body's ability to resist disease. Whenever the lymph system is overwhelmed by these toxic materials, or whenever the lymphatic filters become clogged (especially during illness) the system stores toxic mucous.

The lymph system is similar to the pipes that carry waste in a house. Over time, wastes build up on the insides of the pipe walls and start to clog the system. The same thing happens in the lymph system. Toxic mucous and other wastes build up in the lymph system and hinder its function.

Because the lymph system is a part of the immune system, it is vital that its function not be hindered by useless wastes that can be naturally flushed out. There is a domino effect of good health for the entire body if this system is kept clean and healthy. Otherwise chronic illness of various types can result.

How Can the Lymph System Be Cleansed?

Fortunately, the lymph system can be stimulated to release its wastes in a natural, gentle way, and at the same time to replace its own lymphatic fluids.

The best results are achieved after a full Complex Liver Cleansing. For Lymph Cleansing, the Center uses mineral salt and/or juice therapy, lymphatic massage, and Colon Cleansing. A highly concentrated mineral salt solution consumed in the morning creates a reverse osmosis condition in the body, attracting the old lymph fluids to the mineral salt solution. The old lymph fluids pass through the intestinal walls and are eliminated with the feces and urine. Fresh juices absorb well at this time, and their biologically active water replaces the old and dirty lymph fluids.

What Benefits Will I Receive from a Lymph Cleansing?

- Rejuvenates the white blood cells.
- Stimulates such glands the liver, pancreas, etc.
- Improves digestion.
- Cleanses the kidneys, ureters and joints.
- Increases immunity.
- Helps the body fight diseases.

Who Needs a Lymph Cleanse?

Everyone needs to have his or her lymph system cleansed from all the wastes that have built up over a lifetime. Cleansing this important system of the body helps to cleanse every organ and system you have. The Lymph Cleansing offered by the Center has far reaching health effects because the lymph system reaches into every part of the body.

When Should I Have My Lymph System Cleansed?

The Lymph Cleansing produces the very best results after completing Colon Cleansing, Complex Liver Cleansing, Kidney Cleansing and Small Intestine Cleansing. You will need a minimum of three separate Lymph Cleansings.

Instructions
for
Lymph Cleansing

"Laying the foundation . . .
day of dedication."

In order to maximize the results of Lymph Cleansing, it is necessary first to cleanse the large intestine (colon) and the liver.

However, if personal circumstances do not permit Colon Cleansing and Complex Liver Cleansing to be completed first, then Lymph Cleansing can still be beneficial. In this case it would be best to do the Lymph Cleansing three days in a row, or if necessary every other day for three days.

If one is able to complete Colon and Complex Liver Cleansings before cleansing the lymph, then the time between Lymph Cleansings can be a week or two.

How Many Procedures Are Required for Lymph Cleansing?

The amount of lymphatic and other fluids in the body is approximately twelve liters. During one day of lymphatic cleansing, about four liters of lymphatic fluid are exchanged. (*Lymph fluids have a light yellow and white color. Juices change the color.*) Therefore, full Lymph Cleansing, or full fluid exchange, requires three procedures.

Usually, for maintaining health and preventing disease, Lymph Cleansing should be done once every one to three years, depending on the person's health condition and other cleansing programs. If necessary, Lymph Cleansing can be repeated after one to three months.

Two or Three Days Before the Lymph Cleansing

1. Eat only a vegetarian diet for two to three days prior to Lymph Cleansing with the main accent on fresh fruits and vegetables, freshly made organic fruit and vegetable juices, clean distilled water in large enough amount, whole grains, soups, etc.

2. Take a warm bath once a day for two or three days prior to Lymph Cleansing. Use herbs (sage, camomile) and sea salt in the water, and keep the atmosphere relaxing.

3. Obtain whatever kitchen items you may need such as:
    Citrus juicer - quality is important
    Cutting boards - large, impermeable
    Strainers - the finer the mesh the better
    Large glass or ceramic pitcher (other types can react
        with the juices)

One Day Before the Lymph Cleansing

The citrus fruits you will need are:
- **10-12   organic oranges**
- **8-10   organic grapefruits**
- **5-8   organic lemons**
- **2 liters of clean, distilled water**

Please note that **these are approximate amounts**. You may need more depending on the "juiciness" of the citrus fruits available in your local area. You may also need more depending on your personal body size. Larger persons have more lymphatic fluid and therefore need to replace a larger volume. Also, try to purchase citrus fruits that are medium-sized and properly ripe. (This is a good time to support your local health food grocery store.)

If you are allergic to any of the above citrus fruits, you will have to substitute carrots and celery. In this case you will need to buy:
- 30-40   organic carrots
- 10-20   organic celery sticks
- 2 liters of clean, distilled water

Again, please note that **these are approximate amounts**.

Keep these foods (either citrus fruits or vegetables) at room temperature until use. Also, make ice cubes from the distilled water, or from fresh, organic orange juice or grapefruit juice.

On the Day of the Lymph Cleansing

Clean and organize your kitchen so that nothing will interfere with the healthiness and ease of your preparations.

Put one or two pieces of ice in your distilled water every two or three hours. The physical changes ice undergoes when melting create special properties in the water.

Set out all the kitchen utensils you will need:

- Citrus juicer
- Cutting boards
- Strainers
- Pitcher
- Sharp kitchen knives
- Clean glasses

You will make freshly squeezed citrus juice. The proportion of orange to grapefruit to lemon is 4.5:4.5:1. It is better to make this juice throughout the day as opposed to all at once. This will help retain the vitality of the juices. Also, all of these juices must be strained to remove seeds and pulp. All measurements of juice volume must be done after straining.

Recipe for Biologically Active Drink
for the Renewal of Lymphatic Fluids

10-12 oranges	900 ml. juice	4.5 cups	36 oz.
6-8-10 grapefruits	900 ml. juice	4.5 cups	36 oz.
4-5-8 lemons	200 ml. juice	1 cup	8 oz.
Total:	2000 ml. juice	10 cups	80 oz.

Once this juice has been made, store it in a glass or ceramic pitcher in your refrigerator. **It is important to keep all fresh juices cool and away from light to preserve their vitamins and minerals.** Cover the pitcher tightly with plastic wrap to limit further air circulation inside the pitcher of juice.

Also, do not mix the juices with water until immediately before drinking. Otherwise chemical reactions will occur that will hinder the effectiveness of the juices.

Secondary Recipe for Lymphatic Renewal Drink

30-40 carrots	1500 ml. juice	7.5 cups	60 oz.
10-20 celery sticks	500 ml. juice	2.5 cups	20 oz.
Total:	2000 ml. juice	10 cups	80 oz.

The same recommendations apply to these vegetable juices: both of these juices must be strained to remove pulp, the mixture must be stored in a glass or ceramic pitcher in the refrigerator until use, and do not mix the juices with water until immediately before drinking. *All measurements of juice volume must be done after straining.*

1. **Prepare the juices from the recipe above beginning at 7:00 a.m.** (*Make the juices, strain them, and put them immediately in the refrigerator.*)

2. When you finish making the juices (approximately 8:00 a.m.) **drink the *solution* provided by the Center.** The solution should be kept in the refrigerator as well. Then, before you start, you will warm the solution to body temperature as described for juices below. This solution "jump starts" the cleansing process. If the taste of the solution is unpleasant, take two or three sips of clean water, or suck (*but not swallow*) a piece of orange or grapefruit.

The high concentration of natural salt in the solution creates an osmotic effect in the body (the passage of a "solvent" from a less concentrated to a more concentrated solution through a semipermeable membrane). The highly concentrated salt solution draws to itself the less concentrated fluid—the lymph—through the walls of the digestive system. This solution may also have a laxative effect, so you will want to stay within easy access of a toilet for the morning, and perhaps the afternoon. It will usually take 30 to 45 minutes, sometimes up to two hours, to create the urge to go to the bathroom.

3. Right after drinking the solution, **take a warm bath or shower** for 15 to 20 minutes. The moist heat of the warm bath begins and enhances the process of pulling old lymphatic fluids and associated toxins into the digestive system, through which they are sent to the colon and kidneys.

4. After the warm bath, **begin to drink the cool juice and water** mixture prepared earlier. Mix the juices and the distilled water "fifty-fifty" in the following manner:

    a. Shake the juice container to stir its contents.
    b. Pour 4 oz. (100 g.) of juice into a glass.
    c. Put the container of juice back in the refrigerator immediately.
    d. Pour 4 oz. (100 g.) of distilled water into the glass with the juice.
    e. Warm the juice/water mixture gently to body temperature in a pan of hot water (see below).
    f. Drink it with moderate speed.

5. You should repeat this process every 20-30 minutes until you finish all the juice. If you have not finished all of the juice/water mixture by the time of your appointment at the Center, please bring it with you. You will finish drinking it when you come to the Center.

Important Consideration: Please remember this about the biologically active, diluted juice you are drinking: It is absorbed by the body and exchanged for the old toxic lymph. **These juices are the raw material from which your new lymphatic fluids are made.** Because of this, you want the highest quality fruit (or vegetable) juices possible. **Canned juices or other purchased/prepared juices are biologically dead and filled with artificial ingredients.** Who would want to use such unnatural, pre-poisoned material to create new lymph fluids? Stick with making your own juices from organically grown produce, and making them just before using them. Remember that light and heat damage the vitality of the juices, so put them in the refrigerator to keep them cool and away from light. Also cover the pitcher tightly with plastic wrap to limit further air circulation inside the pitcher of juice.

How to warm the juice/water mixture slowly: Warm water in a pan until it is very warm but not hot. Place the glass containing the juice/water mixture into the warm water. Mix the juice solution periodically with a spoon. Take a drop from the solution periodically, and put on the back of the hand, to check its temperature. **Do not let the juice/water mixture get hot.**

In the first three or four hours, the cleansing will come through the large intestine (colon). Then the process will change, and the cleansing will continue through the kidney in the form of urine.

Services Provided at the Center

1. *Lymphatic Massage (Drainage)* This service is done by using two pieces of state-of-the-art equipment:

a. **GX-99.** This machine uses mechanical vibrations at a frequency of between 30 and 50 millihertz to stimulate the lymph system to release old lymph fluids. The GX-99 helps to clean the lymphatic ducts and activate the flowing of lymphatic fluids in the muscles and internal organs. The use of this machine has at least two side benefits:

- Slimming the body.
- Lessening the cellulite.

You don't have to be enrolled in any program to enjoy the benefits of the GX-99.

b. **LTD-90 ("Lustre").** This machine uses light energy on the tender parts of the body where major lymph nodes are located. The LTD-90 helps to clean the lymph nodes of the neck, armpits, groin, and breast areas. Because the Center has a husband and wife team (with more than a quarter of a century's experience) performing all therapies, clients may elect to have someone of the same gender operate this equipment, or to do it themselves after receiving instruction.

The use of the LTD-90 also has additional benefits:

- Risk reduction for breast cancer.
- Risk reduction for lymph cancer.
- Risk reduction for blood cancer.

You don't have to be enrolled in any program to enjoy the benefits of the LTD-90.

The LTD-90: Dr. DeMonford's machine uses neon light which passes through the skin and causes the molecules of blood and lymph to separate in the lymph system. This eases the transition of the old, toxic lymphatic fluids, relieves soreness in the lymph nodes and increases oxygen flow to prevent tissues from becoming hard.

2. ***Cleansing of the Large Intestine***. The Center uses Colon Cleansing (colon hydrotherapy) to gently flush out the rest of the toxic lymphatic fluids in order to prevent their reabsorption in the colon.

3. ***Infrared Sauna***. The Cleansing Infrared Sauna activates and supports the function of the eliminating organs, such as the liver and kidneys, drawing toxins from the lymph system and the rest of the body, and removing them through the skin by perspiration.

During this day, you probably will not have any desire to eat. But if you feel hungry at the end of the day, it is permissible to eat some oranges or grapefruit (*carrots and celery*). Also, you may drink clean water, or eat a small amount of vegetarian food like fresh salad.

Your Diet Following Your Lymph Cleansing

For the next three days after your Lymph Cleansing, your food must be 80-100% raw. This includes fresh fruits, vegetables, and their juices. Ten to twenty percent of your food could be steamed vegetable, vegetable soups, or cooked whole grains.

Therapeutic Effect of Lymph Cleansing and Lymphatic Drainage

Your Lymph Cleansing will provide you with the following benefits:

- Cleansed lymphatic system.
- Brand-new lymphatic fluids
- Cleansed blood vessels and blood.
- Cleansed kidneys.
- Cleansed skin.
- Increased immunity and resistance to many diseases.
- Improved blood quality.
- Activation of the hormonal glands.
- Improved digestion.

Some Disorders and Illnesses Which Could be Solved with Lymph Cleansing

Swollen lymph nodes, skin problems, high cholesterol, constipation, headaches, colds, sinus problems, weak immune system, chronic fatigue, ...

Step #8

Cell Cleansing

> "The Ph.D. of natural healing, helping you reach optimal health and look younger."

How Do Cells Accumulate Waste?

The organs of the human body are made up of tissues, which in turn are made up of billions of individual cells. When we eat food, the stomach, small intestine, and large intestine digest the food in order to separate nutrients (vitamins, minerals, proteins, etc) from unusable materials (waste). The nutrients are then sent to every part of the body to feed these cells.

As the nutrients are "burned" at the cellular level, waste is created within the cells that (too often) is not completely removed. As time passes and cells are replaced, the waste products are left behind within the tissues of that organ. These toxic wastes poison the cells, weakening them and making them susceptible to illness and disease.

The question now is how to gently coax the body, on a cellular level, to release these wastes and thereby strengthen the immune system. The answer lies in proper fasting, preferably under the supervision of a trained professional who can maximize the health benefits of the fast through centuries-proven techniques.

Solving the Problem

When we stop eating, the body seeks to obtain energy anywhere it can. Since no new sources of energy or food are coming in from the outside, it will search around for what it can consume that is already present on the inside of the body.

The human body is incredibly wise when it comes to healing itself, so it naturally avoids consuming any part of itself that is necessary or useful to its own health. Therefore, it begins by eating or consuming dead cells, dying cells, sick cells, and fat cells first.

With its attention now focused on identifying which cells constitute fuel, it begins to recognize more clearly those cells that it cannot consume and that the body cannot use. "House Cleaning" begins in a vigorous and determined way.

The body begins to dump any unhealthy materials such as toxic mucous, tumor and cancer cells, different kinds of salts, cholesterol, the chemical dregs of any kind of drugs, nicotine, and other stagnated matter which is stored in the tissues and organs. The body also disposes of the unseen toxic weight stored inside.

All cleansings, except fasting, cleanse only the internal surface of the organ and its inner passageways where materials have accumulated in masses of various sizes. While these other (valuable) cleansings remove large percentages of accumulated waste, they are unable to reach into the cellular level. Or shall we say, the regular cleansing "cleans the house," but cellular cleansing "sweeps the corners."

The philosophy (and reality) of this is that all toxins in the body decrease your health. The regular cleansings (described in preceding chapters) get the vast majority of toxins, and therefore will strengthen your immune system, lengthen your life, and improve the quality of life. But with cellular cleansing, the remainder of your body's toxins can be removed, thereby taking your immune system to the zenith of its strength, providing the longest life your body can achieve, and maximizing your quality of life.

Fasting

Fasting, by itself, is not enough to truly cleanse the billions of cells of the body. Although critically important to this procedure, it still needs a little help.

The Center maximizes the natural flushing action of the body during fasting with such techniques as a full body "healing massage," a cleansing sauna, and freshly made natural juices used in correct sequence and amount. During this time, the body is flushed with lots of clean water, while also given strategic, limited nourishment in the form of biologically active juices and organic herbal teas.

When these elements are synchronized under the trained eye of professionals with decades of experience, and tailored for your particular circumstance, the body fully activates the flushing out of toxins down to the cellular level, and with the least discomfort.

Once this process has begun during the fast, the body begins to "eat" its own diseases, harmful bacteria, unhealthy chemicals brought into the body, and toxins created in the body. Parasites that may be present weaken and sometimes die, and are then excreted.

Fasting helps the body to dispose of toxic matter by supporting and cleansing all eliminating organs. The Center, in turn, supports the eliminating organs such as the skin (through Cleansing Sauna), the colon (through Colon Cleansing), and the other internal organs (through Cleansing Massage).

Does This Process Slow Down Aging?

On the cellular level, youth and aging are determined by the relative amount of old and young cells. In youth, the number of young, healthy, and strong cells predominates over the number of old, weak, and sick cells. With time, the cells become polluted and old, and the renewing ability of the body decreases.

During fasting, by switching from outer to inner nourishment, the body "eats" old and sick cells, and the body's ability to exchange old cells for new cells increases and speeds up. Metabolism improves.

During the breaking of the fast (the renewal period), the body replaces the "eaten" cells for new, healthy, young cells. At the Center, the renewal period is accompanied by healthy, specialized eating and special exercises. (Do not underestimate the importance how to break the fast. If done incorrectly, many, if not most, of the benefits of fasting can be destroyed.)

The person who does seasonal fasting regularly, without waiting for disease to come, looks so much younger than his or her age. This person is full of energy and has high resistance to disease.

Which Kind of Fasting Is Used in Our Center?

We use the **Nourishing and Rejuvenative Fasting,** which is the easiest and least stressful kind of fasting.

During this kind of fasting, you will receive a detailed program, which allows you to drink clean water, herbal teas, fresh fruit juices, vegetable juices, and vegetable broth. If done correctly, one may also chew some vegetables without swallowing anything except the juice. (Inquire about Koyfman Fasting©.)

During Fasting, Will a Person Have Enough Energy to Continue Working?

The Nourishing and Rejuvenative Fast puts the body on a high energy level. During the fasting, energy channels open up and become unclogged. Because of this, fasting promotes the body's reception of cosmic, earth, air, and sun energy. Energy is released and received from the "chewing" of the water, and the fruit and vegetable juices, as well as from the chewing only of some vegetables.

Therefore, the energy level of a fasting person is not lower than the energy level of the person who eats. Sometimes it is even higher.

Therapeutic Effects of Fasting

1. Helps to lose visible weight.
2. Cleanses the body on the cellular level.
3. Helps the body to heal itself.
4. Rejuvenates the body.
5. Supports, strengthens, improves the immune system.

6. Increases belief in one's own strength.
7. Cleanses on the emotional and psychological levels.
8. Improves digestion.
9. Improves **metabolism**.
10. Improves vision and hearing.
11. Improves the skin condition.
12. Gives the colon rest during the fast.
13. Activates the work of the colon after the fast.
14. Promotes active and healthy longevity.

Instructions
for
Cell Cleansing

"A program of healing and
rejuvenating fasting."

Preparation for the Fast

**To make fasting successful and yield the best results,
it is necessary to do all the steps properly.**
Three days prior to beginning the fast, stay on a strict
cleansing vegetarian diet: fruits, soaked dried fruits, fresh
fruit and vegetable juices, fresh salads, soups, grains, small
amounts of nuts and seeds soaked in water for 4-8 hours.

Entering the Fast

Often those who don't properly understand the
processes that happen in the body during fasting begin
fasting without any special care or plan, and without the
needed background knowledge. This is not wise.
During fasting, the system does not stop feeding; it
simply reorients its hunger during the fast to internal
feeding. If the fasting begins without complete cleansing of

the digestive system, then the body will spend a long time feeding itself on leftover toxins and thereby poisoning itself. Such fasting is difficult for the person fasting. You may feel weakness, dizziness, nausea, or heart palpitations.

When fasting begins with a full cleansing of the various organs in the body, as described in the preceding chapters, then the body will not (cannot) waste its time and energy consuming toxins. It goes directly to feeding on old/dead/dying/sick cells. These cells go through the digestive process and are "digested" in the sense that what is useful is separated from what is not useful. (The healthy cells are left alone; the digestive process does not touch them.)

As these cells are burned in the fire of internal digestion, what nutrients are available feed the body, and the remainder (toxic mucus, excessive fat, tumors, cancer cells, etc) are sent out of the body via the excretory organs.

During such fasting some people can lose as much as 10 to 70 pounds of toxic weight, depending on personal circumstances. With this load of poisonous weight ("dead weight," pun intended) gone from the body, the healing and rejuvenation processes and shift into fifth gear.

The Role of the Liver in Fasting

The liver, ever the superstar of healing, plays a very important role during the fast. As useless cells are digested, it is the liver that neutralizes the toxins released by the digestion. If, before the fast, the liver is fully cleansed and in tip-top shape, it can better handle the work and make the fast easier to go through. **A day of Complex Liver Cleansing could be an entrance to the fast.**

So, if we combine Complex Liver Cleansing with the cleansing of the whole digestive system (Stomach, Colon

106

and Small Intestine cleansings), fasting will be more effective, and you can go through the fast with ease and comfort. If one can not do all of these cleansings prior to fasting then, at a bare minimum, one should precede fasting with Colon Cleansing.

Important Procedures During the Fast

During the fast, and through the first week after you break the fast, you should consider doing any of the following combinations of procedures. **The more procedures you do the more toxins you expel and the better you feel.**
• Colon Cleansing.
• Colon Cleansing with Internal Organ Massage.
• Colon Cleansing with sauna.
• Full body cleansing massage with a Colon Cleansing and sauna.

Doing the Fast Itself

This is a sample of a fasting schedule during the day. Depending on your personal and work schedule, plus any personal health problems, you can change it. Just keep in mind the main principles. (See section below entitled, "Important Principles of Fasting.")

7:00 a.m.   a.   In the morning after waking up, drink 1 to 2 glasses of warm, distilled water plus 1 tsp. strained lemon juice. Add to the water a pinch of sea salt for neutralizing toxins which accumulate in the stomach during the night.

107

b.	Warm or contrast shower without soap.
c.	Dry skin brush massage, 3 to 5 minutes.
d.	Light morning exercise, 10 to 15 minutes.
e.	Outside walking, 20 minutes to 1 hour, with cleansing breathing technique (described in the book, *Healing through Cleansing,* in the chapter on the lungs).

9:00 a.m.   Big cup of warm herbal mint tea.

11:00 a.m.   Fruit juice: ½ cup juice (citrus, such as grapefruit, lemon, or orange, or apple) in ½ cup distilled water. **All juices on a fast must be strained**. This will prevent the stomach from having to work during the fast by digesting small food particles. It will also help to rest the colon. The juice will be absorbed directly by the small intestines.

1:00 p.m.   Vegetable juice (strained): 1 to 2 glasses.
- 60% choice of 2-3 kinds of green juices: celery, romaine lettuce, spinach, kale, cucumber, mustard and other greens.
- 40% juice from carrots, apples or pineapples.

3:00 p.m.   Warm herbal tea from rose hips or fasting tea.

5:00 p.m.   a.   Apple/beet juice: 4 apples plus 1/4 beet.

b.   1 to 2 glasses clean, distilled water.

7:00 p.m.   1 to 2 cups warm, strained Potassium
                Vegetable Broth. (No substitute broth is
                allowed. See below for recipe.)

9:00 p.m.   Warm herbal tea with camomile. May add ⅓
                to ½ tsp. honey dissolved in tea. If you have
                yeast in your body, do not use honey.

Walking before going to bed, 30 minutes. This is NOT
power walking, but strolling *for relaxation,* so do not walk
too fast.

Warm shower without soap. This is to increase circulation
and not for exterior cleanliness. Shower or bathe for
exterior cleanliness at a different time.

10:00-11:00 p.m.   Go to bed no later than this time.

Recipe for Potassium Vegetable Broth:

Base: 1. Two big organic potatoes cut into cubes (1 cm.).
            2. One glass shredded carrot.
            3. One glass shredded beet.
            4. One glass shredded celery (sticks or root).

Can be added: 1. One-half glass of cut onion.
                        2. Roots of parsley.
                        3. Beet tops.

Cover this with good clean water or previously distilled
water, 1 or 2 cm. above the vegetables.

Bring to a boil, then continue to simmer on low heat for 30 minutes.

Turn off heat.

Add upper green parts of beet, dill and parsley. Let stand for 30 minutes.

Strain.

While it is still warm, drink 1 or 2 eight-ounce cups.

Put the rest in the refrigerator.

Notice: All teas, juices, broths must be strained and warm or cool (never cold) when drunk. Do not eat the solids.

One woman in our Center was in her second three-week fast without receiving the expected benefits in energy and weight loss. We could not understand this until she mentioned that she used cubes of organic chicken broth instead of this recipe. Here are the reasons this is not allowed.

During this healing and rejuvenating fast, one must avoid fats, amino acids, and salt, which are items very present in pre-processed chicken broth, even if organic. Chicken soup may be a homemade remedy that works in certain instances, but this healing and rejuvenating fast follows a different principle of healing.

Further, ridding your body of disease and reversing the aging process are no small accomplishments. The fast that will be effective requires much work and a commitment to be involved in your own healing. **Buying ready-made, pre-processed solutions will never suffice, even if they are organic and vegetable.**

Important Principles of Fasting

1. Wear clean clothes because they will help to accumulate more toxins from the skin. So change your clothes every single day. The underwear is the most important article of clothing here.
2. Use underwear made of natural fibers, not synthetic materials. Synthetic clothes accumulate negative electricity which can destroy body energies.
3. Wear extra clothing to stay warm since you might feel cold during a fast. If you have more clothes and don't feel cold, you save more energy for healing rather than wasting it for heating.
4. Before drinking anything, rinse your mouth with water, or water plus baking soda, or water and lemon juice.
5. During the day, try to find the time for walking 1 to 2 hours. During fasting, our bodies need more oxygen to neutralize the toxins.
6. Do a dry brush massage every morning and possibly every evening for 5-10 minutes.
7. Get some light exercise.
8. Try to stay calm, concentrate on yourself, not reacting to anything around you.
9. Try to find time for resting (not sleeping) with warm water bottle or heating pad on the right side for 30 to 60 minutes to heat your liver. (It will help your liver to detoxify itself and your whole body).
10. At any time, when you feel thirst, hunger or discomfort, drink distilled water.
11. Take a warm bath at least every other day, better every day. During fasting, the body cools down without food to warm it up. A warm bath helps to warm it up, stimulate circulation for toxin removal and to soak the toxins out. If you are doing a warm bath, you may skip #9 above.

12. Call the Center any time you feel you need support or help.
13. Don't break the fast without consulting with the Center. Breaking the fast when you are not feeling well involves a special program.

Tips to Remember

- Fasting cleanses and rejuvenates the whole body down to the cellular level.
- During fasting some people feel a slight discomfort, plus "flashbacks" to the feelings of old diseases and disorders, weakness, etc., as their stored remnants work themselves out. But all of this is for a short period of time, tolerable, and so much easier than the diseases themselves. These are called "healing events."
- If you feel bad, drink a cup of water with a pinch of sea salt to neutralize toxins (people who don't have yeast can add 1/3 teaspoon of honey).
- The benefits fasting brings are so amazing that it is worth the challenge.
- Look at this struggle as your fight with the sickness living inside you. In this fight you must win.

Caution: After you complete your fast, it is very important to break the fast correctly. Incorrect exiting from the fast may destroy all the benefits from your efforts as well as your health.

To find out how to break a fast, read the next chapter entitled, "Detailed Instructions for Exiting the Fast."

Detailed Instructions
for
Exiting the Fast

A Little Wisdom Please

During the fast, your body burned up a lot of old cells. When you start eating again, your body will use this new nutritional material to build new cells that were lost during fasting.

The question here is what level of quality do you want to have?

If you eat organic foods of the highest quality, you will build cells of the highest quality. If you chose to go back to eating processed foods with their burden of toxins built in, then you will get cells that come packaged with toxins. Why lose the ground you just gained?

Caveat Emptor

ATTENTION: The transition from fasting to regular food is very important. Breaking the rules of this transition period can undo all of the benefits and strengths of your fast. In fact, violating these rules can even harm your health.

On the other hand, strictly following these rules during this period will enhance the success of the cleansing therapy.

The Center is not responsible for any problems if you do not strictly abide by the rules found here.

The length of the transition period is equal to the length of the fast.

STRICTLY PROHIBITED AFTER THE FAST

1. Don't use any SALT or any products containing salt.
2. Don't eat *fatty* or *spicy* foods.
3. Don't consume any milk or any milk products.
4. Don't use red meat, fish, chicken, turkey, etc.
5. Don't eat any canned foods.
6. Don't eat *dead foods*: foods that are not natural, that have been processed, that contain artificial ingredients, empty calories, are not fresh, have questionable quality, or are overcooked.
7. Don't eat to fullness. Overeating will produce toxins and make you feel weak and worse. (If you still feel hungry, you ate the right amount.)

STRICTLY EXPECTED PRACTICES FOR EXITING THE FAST

1. Do continue drinking vegetable and fruit juices (freshly made, natural, organic), herbal teas, and filtered water. (Fluids will decrease the feeling of hunger and compensate for the lesser amount of food.)
2. Do chew your food very thoroughly. This is important because chewing (and the mixing of saliva) is the first step in digestion. If an insufficient amount of saliva is mixed and/or food is not chewed thoroughly, then food does not digest fully. Incomplete digestion leads to toxins being formed in the body. This increases the work the digestive system must do, and therefore steals energy from the body.
3. Do continue with the procedures you used during fasting, such as dry-brush massage, walking, warm baths, jumping on rebounder, yoga, resting when tired, intentional relaxation, and light exercise with weights. Exercise with weights and yoga exercises will improve the circulation in muscles and in internal organs, promoting the building inside you of new, young, healthy cells.
4. After the first few days of fasting, the colon has so little in it for stimulation, that in order to keep it working, you will need to do Cleansing Exercises. Two times the first week, still do Colon Cleansing. During the second week, do a Colon Cleansing one time.

Exiting the Fast: A Schedule

First Day   You may skip some of this if you don't feel hungry.

7:00 a.m.	Drink 1 to 2 glasses of distilled water plus 1-2 tsp. strained lemon juice per glass.
9:00 a.m.	Drink the broth from cooked **brown** rice (1 or 2 tablespoons brown rice to 1 quart water.) Cook for about 40 minutes, then strain. *Find a place to sit undisturbed and think of something pleasant because this a very important time for your body, the moment of first food.* Drink the warm broth, **slowly.** Hold each sip in your mouth approximately 15 or 20 seconds. Drink one cup only.
	During this period, new cells are building from the food eaten and from the way this food is assimilated. So, to build up new, young and healthy cells, follow strictly all diet recommendations.
11:00 a.m.	Drink 1 cup warm herbal mint tea. (You may add 1 tsp. of strained lemon juice.)
1:00 p.m.	**Variation #1:** One clean, organic tomato blanched (dipped in boiling water for 10-15 seconds) and peeled; eat very slowly.
	Variation #2: Five or six ounces of plain organic kefir.
3:00 p.m.	Drink one glass of any kind of vegetable juice (freshly made, natural, organic).

5:00 p.m.	**Variation #1:** One clean, organic, green, sour APPLE (*Granny Smith* variety), peeled, cored, shredded; eat very slowly. **Variation #2:** Cooked brown rice soup (no more than 5 ounces, nothing more than rice, no salt, no sugar); eat very slowly; chew a minimum of 50 times.
7:00 p.m.	Drink vegetable broth, no more than 1 cup.
9:00 p.m.	Drink 1 cup camomile tea and 1 tsp. strained lemon juice.
Second Day	**Persons who are underweight** need to take a warm bath daily for the next one to two weeks, and, after the bath, lubricate the skin with warm olive oil, wait 20 minutes, and then take a warm shower.
Breakfast	**Variation #1:** 1 small whole, natural, organic, sour apple (Granny Smith), cleaned and peeled. (One more apple if desired.) **Variation #2:** Whole oat soup: 3 tbs. oats, boiled in 1 quart water for 30 minutes or more, until the oats are soft. Eat no more than 8 oz. or 200 grams, 1 glass.
Lunch	**Variation #1:** Finely shredded carrot (1 to 1 ½ medium carrots, 150 to 200 grams or 5-7 oz.).

Variation #2: Vegetable soup: Cut vegetables into small pieces; put them in already boiling water. Do not overcook; vegetables should still have a "crunch" to them when they are eaten. Do not eat more than 150 grams or 6 oz.

Dinner
Variation #1: Fresh salad (no more than 200 grams or 8 oz. or 1 cup):
Ingredients: shredded carrot, peeled and diced fresh cucumber, soft part of Romaine lettuce.
Dressing: strained juice from lemon, no more than 1 tbs.

Variation #2: Whole oats, cooked until soft, eaten plain, no more than 100 grams or 5 to 6 oz. Don't add any dressing or seasoning.

Third Day
With each meal, eat 1-2 average-sized cloves of garlic for the next 1 to 2 weeks.

Breakfast
Variation #1: 1 sweet, fresh apple, 1 sweet pear, 250 to 300 grams or 10 oz.
Variation #2: 2 sweet apples.

Lunch
Variation #1: Whole brown rice, cooked until soft, eaten plain, 100 to 150 grams or 5 to 7 oz. Don't add any dressing or seasoning.

Variation #2: Fresh salad (200 to 250 grams or 8 to 10 oz.)

Ingredients: 1 shredded carrot, ½ stick diced celery, ½ peeled and diced cucumber. Dressing: strained juice from fresh tomato.

Dinner   **Variation #1:** Homemade vegetable soup, 150 to 200 grams or 8 to 10 oz.

Variation #2: Whole buckwheat or millet, cooked until soft, eaten plain, 100 to 150 grams or 5 to 7 oz. Don't add any dressing or seasoning.

Fourth Day

Breakfast   Two fruits: either two sweet fruits or two sour fruits, but **not** sweet and sour combined. No more than 250 grams or 10 oz.

Lunch   Fresh salad: four kinds of vegetables (carrot, cucumber, celery, lettuce, tomato) with sour dressing of lemon juice, grapefruit juice, or tomato juice.

Dinner   Whole buckwheat plus steamed onions, carrots, and celery, cooked in their own juice. To steam vegetables in their own juice, add a small amount of water to the vegetables in a pan over low heat. The vegetables will release their own juices for cooking. Eat no more than 250 grams or 10 oz.

Fifth Day

Breakfast   Fruits of two or three kinds, but do not mix sweet and sour fruits. No more than 250 to 300 grams or 10 to 12 oz.

Lunch   **Variation #1:** Vegetable soup plus one small, steamed, organic potato. Do not eat more than 300 grams or 12 oz.

     Variation #2: Fresh salad plus one small, steamed, organic potato. Do not eat more than 300 grams or 12 oz.

Dinner   Whole buckwheat or millet or oats or brown rice or quinoa, plus onion, carrot, and celery, cooked in their own juice. Just before eating add 1 tsp. olive oil (organic, cold pressed, virgin). Eat no more than 250 grams or 10 oz.

Day Six through Day Fourteen (General Instructions)

Breakfast   Main food is fresh fruits or dried fruits, soaked in water overnight.

Lunch   Fresh salad with steamed potato or any kind of cooked grains.

Dinner   Vegetable soup, or any kind of grains with vegetables cooked in their own juice. During dinner, you may add to each serving 1 tbs. olive oil.

After two weeks, carefully add new foods: legumes (very well cooked), raw nuts, and sometimes a small amount of fish in correct combination, etc. *Good luck!*

Exiting the Fast with Transition to a Living Food Diet

If you want to go on a living food diet, fasting is the best way to start. Juice fasting in itself is a living food diet, therefore exiting the fast on raw food will be a logical continuation of this diet.

Caution: People who have weak digestion, bloating, and other stomach problems need to choose only those foods which agree with their digestion. When your digestion improves you can gradually introduce new foods and pay attention to how your digestion reacts.

If some food still creates discomfort, you should avoid that food now and try it again later if desired. Possibly during that time your digestion will improve, and then you will be able to eat that food. If not, if it again produces discomfort, indigestion, or gas, then wait.

Don't rush to get all of the vitamins and minerals possible at once. If you try to get the widest variety of food to get more nutrients when your digestion is not ready to handle the variety, instead of nutrients, you will get a large portion of toxins and toxic gases.

However, your body needs nutrition which may not be in the food you eat. Therefore, compensate for this lack of nutrients through fresh juices and liquid vitamins and minerals like Sea Silver or Noni juice.

When you enter the fast with transition to the living food diet, follow the same rules as listed in the first part of this chapter.

Day One

Breakfast   **Fruit Smoothie**
1. In Champion Juicer, make juice from oranges, grapefruit, apples, pineapples, or any two of these in combination.
2. Put pulp through the juicer 2-4 times to make juice thicker and more nutritional.
3. Pour juice into Vita-Mix and add pieces of mango or papaya.
4. Add 3-4 ice cubes made from pure water.
5. Blend 15-30 seconds.
6. If this is too sweet, squeeze some lemon juice into it.
7. Drink.
After breakfast, continue as on fast. Drink juices, herbal tea, and water.

Day Two

Breakfast   Same as Day One.

Lunch   **Vegetable Soup**
1. In Champion Juicer, make juice from carrots and celery.
2. Put pulp through the juicer 1-2 times to make juice thicker and more nutritional.
3. Pour juice into Vita-Mix and add pieces of tomato, cucumber, green pepper, or zucchini, or a combination of 2-3 of these. Juice should always cover the pieces.
4. Blend and drink.
Continue to drink juices, herbal tea, and water as on the fast.

Day Three

Breakfast   **Fruit Smoothie**
Same as Day One, but add to the Fruit
Smoothie half a bunch of spinach in the
blender.

Lunch   **Vegetable Soup**
Same as Day Two, but add to the Vegetable
Soup some kale leaves in the blender.

Dinner   **Vegetable Juice**
In any vegetable juice add 1 tsp. flax seed
oil. Between meals, drink water, herbal tea,
and some juice.

Day Four

Breakfast   **Fruit Smoothie**
Same as Day Three, but add to the Fruit
Smoothie 1-2 Tbs. frozen fruits and 1 tsp.
flax seed oil in the blender.

Lunch   **Vegetable Soup**
Same as Day Three, but add to the Vegetable
Soup 1/3 ripe avocado and 1 medium-sized
clove of garlic in the blender.

Dinner   **Nut Milk**
1. Use 1-2 Tbs. soaked nuts: cashew,
walnut, or others. If almond, it is
recommended to peel the skin.
2. Put nuts into Vita-mix.

3. Add 1 c. apple juice and ½ c. pure water plus 3-4 pitted dates and 3-4 ice cubes.
4. Blend 60 seconds.
5. Strain and chew.

Day Five   Same as Day Four, but add 2 tsp. flax seed oil for breakfast and ½ ripe avocado for lunch.

Day Six

Breakfast   **Fruit Salad**
Cut apples, kiwi, grapes, and put on a plate. Pour over them the Fruit Smoothie made from the recipe on Day Five.

Lunch   **Vegetable Soup**
Cut tomatoes, cucumber, some green onion and bell pepper and pour over the Vegetable Soup made from the recipe on Day Five.

Dinner   **Nut Milk**
Use 2-3 Tbs. nuts that have been soaked 8-12 hours. Blend, strain, and chew the same as on Day Four.

Day Seven through Day Ten

Continue the same as on Day Six.

Then you can carefully add other foods and pay attention to the reaction of your digestion.

Good luck!

Some Disorders and Illnesses Which Could Be Solved with Cell Cleansing

Chronic Fatigue, asthma, allergies, colds, skin problems, enlarged prostate, sexual disorders, digestive problems, weak immune system, insomnia, liver problems, fibroids, tumors, ...

Other Important Services*

. . . at the Koyfman Center

This chapter will give an overview of cleansing services related to the eight steps described so far in this book. These services include:

- Weight Loss Cleansing Program

- Cleansing from Negative Emotions

- Cleansing the Whole Digestive System

- Lung Cleansing

- Thyroid Cleansing Program

- Prostate Cleansing Program

Weight Loss Cleansing Program

When properly and thoughtfully followed, this weight loss program will help you to lose unwanted and unhealthy weight without drugs or other chemicals and their unwelcome side effects. The weight loss program discussed here is not a "diet," and therefore avoids the inconsistent and sometimes harmful results that come from what is often hawked on television, etc.

How Many Pounds Do Toxins Weigh?

Many weight loss programs focus on losing excess fat. To accomplish this, they suggest various methods to burn fat, such as:
- intensive exercise without medical control (overweight people often have heart problems),
- pills which allow you to "eat everything and not gain weight,"
- pills which suppress your appetite, and
- fat-free diets where fats are artificially removed from foods making them more dangerous than the fat itself.

These methods play on only one aspect of losing fat, and then push that one aspect to the extreme. For example, some methods use excessive exercise without taking nutrition into account properly. Others starve the body by the use of chemicals that suppress the appetite. (Some of these hunger suppressing pharmaceuticals are not far removed from some illegal street drugs.) The list goes on.

These unbalanced techniques are too often dangerous. Sometimes (rarely) people have died from these diets or programs. More often their health suffers because after they finish losing the desired weight, they go back to the same old habits that caused them to be overweight in the first place. They regain the lost weight rapidly, and this "whiplashes" the body. This does more harm to both physical and emotional health than the temporary benefits of weight loss.

Worst of all, these artificial weight loss programs ignore a very simple but vital fact: There are two different types of excess weight: excess fat and toxic weight.

A very significant percentage of excess weight in the average person living in the industrialized world is not fat at all; it is toxic weight. This weight accumulates in the internal organs such as the large intestine, the liver, the kidneys, the lymph glands, the small intestine, joints and the stomach. These wastes come packaged in many forms with various compositions. They include colon stones, toxic mucus, liver and gall stones, toxic bile, kidney stones, toxic lymph fluids, and uric acids, to name a few.

As if this were not bad enough, add to this toxic brew the weight and wastes of parasites. Some modern people scoff at the notion that they could have parasites, but the overwhelming evidence, and the indisputable testimonies of the highest ranking national medical professionals make it clear that this is not strictly a

130

phenomenon of Third World countries. It is prevalent here in the United States. (See the chapter on Parasite Cleansing in my book, *Deep Internal Body Cleansing*.)

Parasites thrive on toxins accumulated in the body. After eating such toxins, they excrete new, even more dangerous toxins and gases. For some people these gases accumulate in tissues and can make a person feel and look bloated.

While it is true that excess fat is bad for your health, toxic weight (and parasites) pose a worse problem in terms of excess weight. For example, on the walls of the large intestine alone anywhere from 20-70 pounds of toxic weight can accumulate. This is the weight we need to get rid of first. Additionally, toxic weight which accumulates on the walls of our organs and cells is weight which provides the foundation of disease.

When you get rid of the weight of toxins, you get rid of the weight of your diseases.

What Organs Do We Need to Cleanse to Get Rid of Toxic Weight?

Toxins come into the human system in several different ways, through breathing (inhalation), through eating and drinking (ingestion), and through the skin (absorption). Rarely do toxins enter through injection. Of these different pathways into the body, the most likely route is an improper diet.

Each organ is affected differently, depending on the toxins, the route of entry, and the diverse chemistry in the individual body. Regardless of individual differences, the fact remains that toxic weight accumulates in the organs of our bodies. Which organ is affected more than another depends on personal circumstances.

The colon (large intestine) is the main sewer of the body, and logically accumulates the largest amount of toxic weight. The other digestive organs, the stomach, and the small intestine, are also impacted.

It is also easily understood that the organs that filter out chemical and microscopic biological toxins (the liver and the kidneys) are also heavily contaminated. Like any other filter, they become clogged with time and usage. As they do their work, toxic weight builds up in these critical organs.

The lungs and sinuses are in direct contact with our polluted environment. As such they get "dosed" with airborne contaminants ranging from dust mites, to chemicals from sprays, to vehicle exhaust, to bacteria and viruses. These can physically clog the respiratory system or cause allergic reactions (allergies).

Toxic weight can also be found on the walls of blood vessels, in lymph and lymph nodes, in the pancreas, and in each cell.

Cleansing Leads to Weight Loss, Which Leads to Healing

Deep body cleansing, along with following the principles of healthy eating and a healthy lifestyle, not only lead to losing weight, but also help to heal the body from disease and to rejuvenate the body. This is because, as toxins are cleansed from the body, the metabolism normalizes and helps the body to burn fat the way it is supposed to.

How Much Time Will It Take to Lose Weight Through Cleansing?

On an average, losing weight through "modern" diets takes an advertised 30 days. Unfortunately, in even less time your weight comes back even more than it was before. In addition, there could be new health problems.

On the other hand, losing weight through deep internal body cleansing, as described in this book, does take longer. The difference is that its moderate speed helps to make it safer and longer lasting. The fact that this kind of natural weight loss is really a lifestyle and not a fad means that you will keep the excess fat off for as long as you maintain the lifestyle.

Just as each organ in your body is different in size, shape, and weight, so the cleansing of each of these different organs removes differing amounts and types of toxic weight. You lose the most toxic weight when you cleanse the colon, lymph, liver, and cells.

The very best results come from a combination of cleansing, eating a "living food" diet, and exercise. For 2-6 months, you may lose from 30-100 pounds of toxic weight cleansed from the internal organs as well as "toxic fat." With such an approach you not only lose weight, you look better, have more energy, and in general feel yourself reborn.

Notice: With such a method of losing weight, the skin regains its shape and elasticity, leaving no wrinkles from being overweight.

Therapeutic Benefits of Weight Loss with the Cleansing Method

- Eliminates unpleasant smells from skin (You don't need to use deodorant any more.)
- Improves skin and skin color
- Better sleep
- Improves concentration
- More energy and stamina
- Normalizes blood pressure
- Eliminates pain from joints and back
- Improves vision
- Increases flexibility
- Increases clarity of the mind (Some have said the mind works like a computer after this cleansing.)
- During 6-10 months of cleansing procedures and healthy lifestyle, you lose not only weight but also 10-15 years of biological aging.

Cleansing from Negative Emotions

Cleansing your body, mind, heart, soul, and spirit from negative emotions will provide a surprising boost to the other cleansings, and to overall health status.

Cleansing Number One

Cleansing the body from negative emotions is one of the most important cleansings. In many cases, without this cleansing other cleansing procedures give only temporary results.

Because negative emotions accumulate not only in the physical body (organs, muscles, blood vessels, nerves, and other tissues) but also in the energy field, we need to do cleansing on all levels.

In our Center we start cleansing from negative emotions with physical cleansing procedures. Such an approach gives quick improvement of general conditions and the client becomes more capable of doing other methods of cleansing from negative emotions by himself or herself.

How Negative Thoughts and Emotions Affect the Body

Frequently repeated negative thoughts and emotions can cause tension in muscles and organs so that they tighten up like a frightened animal trying to hide from danger. After the stress has passed, these tensions do not completely disappear but leave behind a "residue" of stress. Unfortunately, these residues can build up with each significant incident.

Problems from this build-up of tension take several different forms. For example, the tension in muscles and organs uses up some of the energy of the body, weakening its immune system. This constant but low-grade tension also contributes to blockages that hinder the circulation of nutrients, blood, lymph, oxygen, energy, etc.

Stress from negative emotions promotes an increased secretion of hormones into the blood. In natural stress situations, such as "fight or flight" physical danger, a person uses up these hormones through increased physical activity such as running, fighting, or working. These hormones are burned up by the muscles, and do not cause harm.

However, in today's social settings, negative emotions are usually not acted upon physically. Therefore, your anger stays inside of you. The large amounts of hormones secreted— instead of being burned off by muscles or used in digestion— attack and harm various organs.

Suppressed or unrealized emotions are the reason for the unbalance in different organs.

More information about negative emotions and cleansing the body from them can be read in Books 2 and 3 of my series, *Healing through Cleansing,* and in my book, *Deep Internal Body Cleansing.*

Cleansing Method to Eliminate Negative Emotions

- Stomach Cleansing
- Complex Liver Cleansing
- Small Intestine Cleansing
- Fasting

Therapeutic Benefits of Cleansing from Negative Emotions

- Eliminate fear, anger, jealousy, etc.
- Make you calm, relaxed, and peaceful.
- Make you balanced.
- Give you more confidence.
- Make you feel secure.
- Make you think positively.
- Give you feelings of hope.
- Make you feel happy.
- Improve your defense against diseases.

Cleansing the Whole Digestive System

Cleansing the whole digestive system in one focused effort will release the body's energies for use in more important matters.

The Kitchen of the Human Body

The digestive system is one of the main channels through which nutrients enter the body. At the same time it is also the main elimination channel. An improper and unhealthy lifestyle transforms the digestive system from a source of nutrients, energy, and health into a source of toxicity, parasites, and illnesses.

The digestive system is the kitchen of the human body, and as such should be the cleanest place in the body. Instead, it becomes like a sewage holding tank full of poisons.

On the positive side, the digestive system is a unique set of organs which has a door on each end. Because the whole body is interested in nutrients, the digestive system has connection with all organs and cells through blood vessels, lymph, and various ducts. These facts present a unique opportunity not only to cleanse and improve the digestive system but also to use it as the main elimination channel through which to cleanse many other organs from toxicity and parasites.

Notice: Details of how to cleanse the whole digestive system will become familiar to the client during the individual consultation.

Why Is Colon Cleansing Not Enough?

Colon Cleansing is a powerful procedure which eliminates toxins and parasites from the large intestine, and greatly improves its function of the colon and the well being of the whole body.

Unfortunately, many people have colons that are in such poor health that its malfunctioning undermines the whole digestive system. Once this starts, a badly impacted colon results in poor digestion that affects the whole digestive system. This causes the colon to be more severely impacted. It is a viscous circle.

So it is important to cleanse and improve the function of all the organs which are involved in digestion: stomach, pancreas, liver, and all parts of the small intestine. When we cleanse the digestive system from toxicity, it stops poisoning the body and improves its nourishment.

What Should I Eat During the Cleansing Procedure?

Diet plays an important role in maintaining health. At the same time, a healthy diet is an agent of cleansing, nourishing, and healing.

Important principles of healthy eating, simple recipes, and weight loss programs are described in Book 4 of my series, *Healing through Cleansing Diet.*

Therapeutic Benefits of Cleansing the Whole Digestive System

- Cleanse and improve stomach function
- Cleanse and improve pancreas function
- Activate the liver
- Partially cleanse and improve the function of the small intestine
- Cleanse and improve the function of the colon
- Cleanse waste from the walls of the whole digestive system
- Eliminate a bad smell from the skin, breath, urine, and bowel
- Eliminate toxic gases
- Activate nerves, digestive buds
- Dramatically improve digestion

Short List of Disorders Which Could Be Helped with this Cleansing

- Constipation
- Poor Digestion
- Chronic Fatigue
- Diabetes
- Obesity
- Chronic Colitis
- Chronic Appendicitis
- Headaches

- Poor Sleep Patterns
- Skin Disorders
- Sexual Disorders
- Use this cleansing to improve your immunity to many diseases.

Preparation for Cleansing the Whole Digestive System

Before Cleansing the Whole Digestive System,
do not eat for 4-6 or more hours.
Your last meal should be light and of a small amount.

Lung Cleansing

Koyfman Center Lung Cleansing is designed to have far-reaching results throughout the whole body.

Weak Lungs - Poor Health

Of all of the "nutrients" that we need for life, air is the most important because its absence will kill you sooner than an absence of food or water. The lungs are also important for nourishing and cleansing the blood cells and all the organs.

Lungs can be weakened by such things as toxic mucus, tobacco residues, airborne chemicals, bacteria and viruses, and a host of other contaminants. The success of any cleansing offered by the Center may well rest upon the health of the lungs.

Lung Cleansing includes cleansing not only the lungs themselves but also the entire air passageway which leads to the lungs: the branchiae, sinuses, and nasal passages.

Who Needs Lung Cleansing?

Practically everybody needs Lung Cleansing and the improvement of lung function, especially
- People who work in unclean air with chemicals, spray paint, and other sprays
- Those who smoke now or did so previously
- Those who have poor digestion
- Those who frequently catch colds and flu
- Those who have allergies, asthma
- Those who have a weak heart
- Those who have depression, frequent stress, weak immune systems and chronic fatigue.

What Is Lung Cleansing?

In my system any cleansing procedure consists of two parts. One part is the part you do yourself described in the series of four books, *Healing through Cleansing*. I recommend these books to everybody who is interested in improving his or her health.

The second part is the part you do at our Center with professional help. Lung Cleansing in our center includes cleansing the whole digestive system which is the main channel by which to eliminate toxins from the body because the digestive system has connections with all other parts of the body.

During the cleansing we utilize techniques which dilute toxins in the lungs, branchiae, and sinuses, and then pull them to the stomach. From the stomach they go to the small intestine, then to the colon and then out.

Notice: *The client receives more detailed information about Lung Cleansing during the individual consultation in our Center.*

Cleansing the lungs is a simple procedure which yields a great result.

Therapeutic Benefits of Lung Cleansing

- Greater immunity to colds and allergies
- Improved digestion
- Increased oxygen nourishment for cells and organs
- Improved blood quality
- Reduced amount of toxins in the body
- Heart function strengthened
- Normalized blood pressure
- Nervous system relaxed and calmed

Short List of Disorders Which Could Be Helped with this Cleansing

- Asthma
- Colds
- Sinus Problems
- Allergies
- Depression
- Digestive Disorders
- Sleep Disorders
- Heart Problems
- Breathing Difficulties
- Weakened Immune System

Thyroid Cleansing Program

The thyroid gland is so small it is often overlooked in considering one's personal health program. The Koyfman Center Thyroid Cleansing Program gives this gland its due place.

King of Glands

The thyroid gland is a little butterfly-shaped organ at the base of the neck that puts out a teaspoon of hormone a year. This hormone affects the metabolism and acts as cellular carburetor for every cell in the body—from the hair follicles down to the toenails.

If the thyroid gland is functioning properly, it acts as a fortress which defends our bodies from the invasion of illness. If the function of the thyroid gland is abnormal or impaired, it can lead to a variety of emotional and physical disorders.

What Is the Reason for Impairment of the Thyroid Gland?

Each organ and gland receives its nutrients from the blood.

If the liver is overloaded with toxins it will not be able to cleanse the blood, and toxins or poisons will spread throughout the body via the blood vessels and lymph. In this case the thyroid gland gradually accumulates toxins on its surface. As these toxic deposits thicken, they eventually block the path by which the thyroid gland receives nutrients.

Iodine is the number one nutrient for the thyroid gland. If the fluids we drink and the foods we eat don't have enough of this mineral, the function of the thyroid gland can become impaired.

What Health Problems Can Be Created by an Impaired Thyroid Gland?

Thyroid dysfunction may cause:
* Weakness
* Dry Coarse Skin
* Slow Speech
* Coarse Hair
* Hair Loss
* Weight Gain
* Difficulty Breathing
* Problems with Menstruation
* Nervousness
* Heart Palpitations
* Severe Chronic Fatigue
* Depression

When the thyroid isn't working properly, the immune system is impaired and this sets up a vicious cycle.

How to Cleanse and Restore the Function of the Thyroid Gland

To cleanse the thyroid gland one must first lay a very powerful foundation. One must first cleanse several of the more important organs before this tiny organ can be reached.

- Cleanse the whole digestive system. This is a foundational procedure to open the main channel to eliminate toxins and stop their spreading.
- Completely cleanse the liver.
- Cleanse the blood and lymph systems.
- Begin to eat healthfully, using green fresh juices which dilute toxins in the thyroid gland.
- Do exercises which activate circulation and restore function in the thyroid gland.

Notice: Diet, exercise, and special thyroid massage are described in Book 2 of my series, *Healing through Cleansing.*

Therapeutic Benefits of Improved Thyroid Gland Functioning

- Sense of Strength
- Soft, Smooth Skin
- Improved Speech Patterns
- Healthy, Flowing Hair
- Possible Thickening of Hair
- Stabilized Weight
- Efficient Breathing
- Ease in Menstruation
- Calmness
- Heart Regularity and Rhythm
- More Energy
- Sense of Well Being and Hope

Prostate Cleansing Program

Prostate Cleansing at the Koyfman Center may be your ticket to refreshing relief and pleasant results.

Male Power

The prostate gland, located just below the bladder, is approximately the size of a walnut. It wraps around the urethra. The prostate generates seminal fluid, which is essential for the survival of sperm. This important gland also lubricates the urethra to prevent infection and promote sperm flow.

Do Not Be Ignorant

Most men are likely to ignore their prostate until it gives trouble. Unfortunately in modern Western society, the majority of prostates are trouble-makers to some degree. Many men are susceptible to the beginnings of prostatic hyperplasia, also known as enlarged prostate.

Age and Prostate Problems

As a man gets older, the cells in his prostate are more likely to multiply, increasing the size of the gland. At the age of 30, a man has only 10 percent chance of having an enlarged prostate. At the age of 60 a man has more than 50 percent chance of having this problem, and more than 90 percent at age 85.

What Are the Symptoms of Prostate Trouble?

Symptoms characterizing an enlarged prostate are:
- Difficulty in starting to urinate
- Increased urinary frequency
- Nighttime trips to the bathroom
- Reduced force of volume of urination
- Sleep deprivation is common among men with prostate trouble.

How to Cleanse the Prostate and Improve Its Function

- Cleanse your whole digestive system (5-10 times) with FIR on the prostate area. Do parasite cleansing for at least 3 months.
- Start eating a healthy diet (read Book 4 in my series, *Healing through Cleansing Diet.*
- Cleanse your small intestine (2-4 times).
- Cleanse your liver (3-5 times).
- Do cell cleansing for 2-3 weeks, three cycles.
- Maintain you colon cleanse and healthy lifestyle forever.

Therapeutic Benefits of Prostate Cleansing

- Better urinary start, force, and volume
- Normalized urinary frequency
- Sleep with less interruption
- More efficient sleep
- Improved sexuality

Maintenance Program

"Do not lose the ground you have gained"

What Have You Achieved after Completing the Eight Steps of the Program?

If in the past you have had a complete cleansing course, or even part of the cleansing program, you are already beginning to notice great improvements in your health. You are definitely interested in maintaining and multiplying your achievement.

1. You feel stronger.
2. You have more energy.
3. Your immune system is stronger and not wasting energy on neutralizing toxins.
4. Your skin looks and feels better.
5. Your breathing is easier and cleaner (no odor).
6. Your large intestine eliminates regularly.
7. You significantly reduced your health age and the health problems which come with age.
8. And much more.

What Is Important to Remember?

The health improvement you have achieved carries with it **no warranty to protect forever** from disorders, illnesses, tiredness, and other problems. Why? We all live in a poisoned world, so our bodies are being polluted continually and constantly. **There is a mistaken opinion that the system can clean itself completely by itself, but if this were possible humans would never get ill and never die.**

Negative emotions can change the chemical make up of the best food products, turning them into poison. Negative emotions also weaken the functions of all eliminating organs. This results in additional pollution of the body.

Food is very important for all of us. Many people eat three times a day. So let's take a look at how the body is polluted from food. The level of pollution from food depends on many factors:

1. Whether it is organic or regular.
2. Whether it is fruit or meat.
3. Whether you have strong or weak digestion.
4. Whether or not you feel hungry when you eat.
5. How you chew your food.
6. The volume you eat
7. The time when you eat, late evening or allowing time to digest the food
8. Whether it is processed food or fresh.

Because we cannot take everything into consideration, let's look at some of the moderating factors. All the volume (100%) of each meal can be divided into three parts.

1. Since the body can assimilate or digest only liquid, therefore, only 15-25% of the volume eaten will be

digested. **Explanation:** Juice made in a juice maker (excluding watermelon, cucumber, and other especially juicy products) may reach one-third (30%) of the full volume, however, this extent of "digestion" or pulverization will not be possible in the presence of poor chewing, bad or missing teeth, or a weak digestive system. So the body gets less juice from eating food than the juice maker gets.

2. The second and third parts together make up approximately 75-85% of the volume eaten. The second part, mostly fiber at 25-40%, is eliminated after 12-36 hours by the work of the colon. The other 25% to 35% of the second part stays longer and cannot be eliminated by colon work alone but depends on the help of pressure from new material pushing, and gravity pulling, on the material inside the colon. This longer time period allows for the process of putrefaction and decay, and the immune system must waste energy to neutralize the poisons produced.

3. The third part is excessive fat, mucous, and non-digestible protein, amounting to 3-10% and more. This is encrusted material that sticks to the colon wall and stays in the system a long time or maybe forever. It becomes dehydrated and pressed to the walls. In time, with lack of oxygen, and with warmth and darkness, this material begins putrefaction and decay, creating an environment for parasites to develop. **If you do preventive Colon Cleansing once in two to four weeks, this will save you from accumulating poisons and parasites.**

Can Regular Preventive Colon Cleansing Completely Protect a Person from All Health Problems?

Even though you try to follow all suggestions and rules of good diet, healthy lifestyle, and cleansing procedures, in reality it is rare that you will do it perfectly. Sometimes you will experience headache, tiredness, colds, stomach discomfort, etc. It is very important **to notice the feeling of the beginning of these disorders,** before they develop.

If you want to solve the problem quickly, you have to stop eating for three to five days, and every other day do some Colon Cleansing. This will quickly help to increase the effectiveness of the immune system and eliminate the problem. The disease will not be able to go deep into the body and do its damage.

We can call them **entrance disorders** if we catch them when they enter, and if you take correct measures in time you will not allow these problems to go inside the system. But if you delay and allow the problem to develop, it can go deep into organs and tissues and cells, and then the problem will continue developing from inside.

Such disorders we can call **internal or chronic disorders.** To solve these problem is very difficult. If they continue a long time these chronic disorders can accumulate and transform into serious illnesses.

Tips to Remember

1. Do not insult others, and try to understand and forgive those who insult you. Insults could be lessons for your own improvement.

2. Try to follow all suggestions about the cleansing diet.

3. Every day do exercises for spine, joints, internal organs, and the endocrine system. If you do your exercises correctly together with outdoor walking, you will activate the **process of cell feeding and cleansing.**

4. Cleanse regularly your colon once in two to four weeks.

5. If you feel the first sign of disorders, stop eating for one to five days, and every other day cleanse your colon.

6. Do Small Intestine Cleansing every three months.

7. Do Complex Liver Cleansing one or two times per year.

8. More often than usual, do specific cleansings which manage your individual problems.

9. If you are interested to get the highest level of health, do a long fast for 2-4 weeks every year, strictly following the instructions in the chapter on cell cleansing.

Other Health Items

Available through Dr. Yakov Koyfman

Order from:

Koyfman's Center for Health and Rejuvenation, Inc.
300 Merchant's Drive, Suite 304
Norcross, Georgia 30093
(770) 908-2305
www.koyfmancenter.com

Cleansing Exercises Posters, $2.50.

Unique Method of Colon Rejuvenation, 95 pages. $10 plus shipping and handling.

Our bodies need constant help eliminating toxic substances which enter the system every day. Daily practice of the rising and restroom exercises described in this book strengthens colon muscles so that, with time, elimination will accompany each meal and eject more toxins than are retained. Also included are principles and recipes for healthy eating, raw meals, and safe cooking technology.

Healing through Cleansing, Books 1-4, 115 pages each. $12 each, plus shipping and handling.

Every day, toxic substances enter our bodies from our environment and form within us due to lifestyle choices and bacterial guests. Our excretory organs need constant, conscious support to cope. How can you help your organs become free of toxins and sustain the health of your entire body? You will find the answers in the pages of this and subsequent books in the Koyfman Series.

Deep Internal Body Cleansing, 152 pages. $15 plus shipping and handling.

If you search for healing and real health, then here you will find answers to your questions Here is information about toxicity and the immune system, healthy eating and eliminating parasites. Here are answers to help you resist hurtful cravings and negative emotions. You really can get health and gain energy through cleansing your body.

Equipment for Use with the Cleansing Exercises

Slant Board, $200.

Specially Designed Foot Rest, $40.

Koyfman's Center for Health and Rejuvenation is located in Norcross, Georgia.

Koyfman's Center for Health and Rejuvenation, Inc.
300 Merchant's Drive, Suite 304
Norcross, Georgia 30093
(770) 908-2305
www.koyfmancenter.com